FIRST AID FOR CATS AND DOGS

This publication is not intended as a substitute for you getting in touch with your vet immediately if your pet is in distress.

It is intended purely to gain you some extra life-saving seconds while you get in touch with your vet.

(Front cover photograph and

internal photographs courtesy Pixabay.com)

Edward Moss

ISBN: 9798399418117

TABLE OF CONTENTS

Important - please read carefully 5
A First Aid kit for your pet 6
Suggested contents for your pet First Aid kit 9
Human medicines 13
Dealing with dosages and scaling them down 17
Human medicines that can be used for pets 17
A basic summary pet responsiveness chart 22
A basic health assessment of your pet 24
Pain in pets 27
Triage 30
Capillary refill time 33
Preventing problems 47
Feed your pet correctly 53
Zoonoses 63
The basics 66
Artificial respiration and CPR (cardiopulmonary 73
resuscitation)
Cardiopulmonary Resuscitation (CPR) 78
How to clean wounds 83
Bandaging techniques 85
Summary list of symptoms and their potential 105
cause/s
Appetite and eating 106
Behaviour 106
Digestion and elimination 109
Ears 111
Eyes 112
Head injuries 113
Head, mouth, nose, and teeth 113
Heart and circulation 117

Rear and tail   117
Legs, hips, and paws   118
Reproductive system   121
Respiratory system   122
Skin and coat   124
Whole-body symptom   127
Emergency procedures   130
Special situations to be aware of   146

- A summary list of common visual signs of symptoms your pet may exhibit begins on page 105

- Please refer to the index at the back of this book for more detailed page references. This should be your port of call for symptoms. But please, do consult your vet – the content of this book is to only help you identify symptoms and provide extra, valuable minutes to contact your vet.

IMPORTANT – PLEASE READ CAREFULLY

It is very important to be ready for any emergency that may threaten your family pet's well-being. They are part of your family.

However, please remember that First Aid is only what it 'says on the tin', that is, the first step you take towards safeguarding the health and well-being of your pet. First Aid simply affords you some extra time to get in touch with your vet.

First Aid is not, and should not, in any way, be seen as a replacement for curing a medical ailment. Neither should it be used as a substitute for the professional medical services of a qualified vet.

Your pet cannot tell you precisely what is wrong with them, and similarly, you are not qualified to make that decision yourself. You can only help, and that is what First Aid is all about.

You **MUST** get your pet to the vet as soon as you can, unless it is something totally superficial (a rose thorn in the side of the leg, for example) that you are 100% confident does not need the **immediate** attention of a vet.

You must never make medical assumptions on behalf of your pet's health unless you are medically qualified to do so. No responsibility can or will be accepted for you solely taking suggestions from this book and NOT contacting your vet.

A First Aid kit for your pet

First aid for dogs and cats, just as it is for humans, is simply what it says.

It is all about responding immediately to an emergency happening that might otherwise seriously impact the health and well-being of your pet. It's all about having the ability, knowledge and "tools" to make a very speedy response. You may not otherwise have time to call the vet (which you need someone to do in tandem with your First Aid treatment) or have the time to search for the precise remedy required.

Most probably on top of all this, you won't possess the correct set of "tools", and the years of training a vet has enables them to fully apply the correct procedure and/or prescribe and administer the correct medicines required.

You simply need to be ready to treat those spur-of-the-moment injuries that can happen at any time. You can most certainly buy ready-prepared First Aid kits containing all the essential basic First Aid care items you may need from either pet stores or the internet.

The warning is to always take care when buying from the internet – for example, the online description of a "wide" bandage may not necessarily be as "wide" as you might otherwise think from reading the description.

Unless you purchase from a recognised reputable source, the contents may contain, unintentionally or otherwise, cheaper substitutes.

If you do decide to assemble your own First Aid kit, you will find following a list of items you should gather together and place in your First Aid kit.

Remember to place any First Aid kit in a dry, accessible place!

Many of the items you need can be obtained from your vet, a specialist pet supply shop, your local pharmacy or even from your local supermarket. Individual items can also be bought from the internet, but as with ready-assembled kits, do check carefully.

As already mentioned, things sometimes are not what they either appear or are stated as being, especially when proprietary brands are stated and you end up receiving generic alternatives. If using the internet, make sure it's a recognised supplier with plenty of positive feedback.

There is one basic constituent in particular that you have to be careful with. Some human disinfectants are wholly unsuitable for use on pets. Your vet can advise you regarding a suitable disinfectant you may wish to keep handy. Also, it is no harm in showing your vet the list of contents, as some may suggest the exclusion or inclusion of some items.

It is a very good idea to label your box **'Pet First Aid Kit – not for other uses'**, so that you have a full kit always at the ready when needed.

This is useful, for example, when you have someone looking after your pet for you. They can then rest assured that they have everything they may need to hand in one place and won't need to go searching for items should they need to seek vet advice on the phone in your absence.

You may also care to have a few items in the car if you regularly travel about with your dog (or with your cat – some breeds of cat do love a trip out).

By so doing, you can not only help your own pet, but you can come to the First Aid of other people's pets if needed.

However, if you do plan to take your pet abroad, the rules, in particular, relating to trips to and from the EU, have changed now that the UK has left the EU.

See here for more details - https://www.gov.uk/taking-your-pet-abroad

When taking a pet out in the car, you should always have a bottle of water and a drinking bowl with you. For those warmer days, also take a towel that you can soak in cold water to use as a body cooler if needed. If you can take a flask of ice, this can be very helpful.

Dogs can become dangerously overheated in the hot weather - brachycephalic (short-nosed) dogs such as French Bulldogs more easily so. This can occur even while travelling in the interior of an air-conditioned car in hot weather.

A clean, strong blanket on which an injured pet can be carried is also a suggested addition.

Suggested contents for your pet First Aid kit

Firstly, you need to have a note pad and pencil in your First Aid kit. In this notebook, you should have the contact name and address of your regular vet, telephone number, mobile number, email address, regular address, times of opening, any emergency numbers and/or any out of hours telephone numbers.

It can also be useful to have the dog's weight, previous illnesses and any treatments (previous or emergency) recorded and the telephone number of a taxi company in case there is a transport problem.

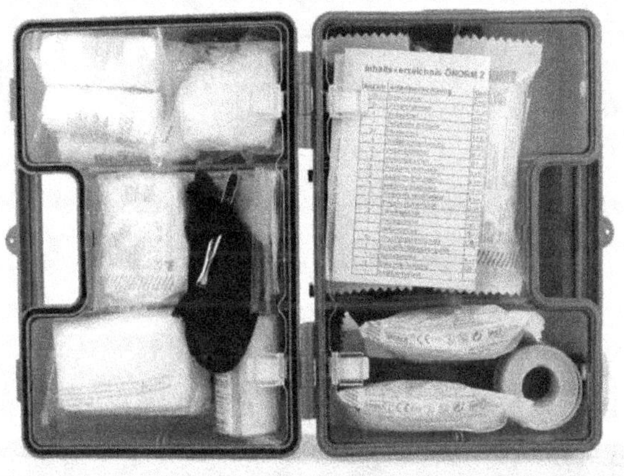

Please note that this is a somewhat "enthusiastic" list, so do check with your vet who might suggest some of the contents are unnecessary or others may need adding or substituting.

Remember, there is absolutely no substitution for that of the professional expert advice from your vet.

- 5cm (2-inch) crepe bandage.
- 5cm and 10cm (2-inch and 4-inch) open-weave cotton bandage.
- A medical bandage that sticks to itself as more layers of it are wound around.
- Antacid emulsion for indigestion and flatulence **only as advised by your vet.**
- Anti-flea spray, **as advised by your vet.**
- Antihistamine tablets – **only as advised by your vet in case of insect stings.**
- Antiseptic. TCP is ideal. Check with your vet if you intend to keep any other type of antiseptic in your kit.
- Bottle of saline solution is also useful for flushing out wounds.
- Bubble wrap. Can be useful for making an improvised splint.
- Cling film – a small roll can be useful for sealing wound areas.
- Cotton wool.
- Ear drops and eye drops **only as advised by your vet.**
- Environmental flea spray.
- Glucose powder **only as advised by your vet.**
- Liquid paraffin for constipation **only as advised by your vet.**
- Meat tenderiser. Soothes wasp and bee stings, mosquito bites and non-poisonous **ONLY** spider bites.

- Nail clippers.
- Roll of two-inch or 3-inch (7.5cm) wide adhesive plaster.
- Shampoo specifically made for dogs. Do not use human shampoos and certainly do not even consider dish-washing liquid.
- Small curved and small sharp straight scissors to cut the coat from around a wound. You may also consider keeping a small nurse's bandage scissors that has a rounded tip on one of the blade ends).
- Small empty bottle for giving liquid medicine.
- Small jar or plastic pot for faeces sample.
- Small nuggets of washing soda. (This acts as an emetic but **should only be used on veterinary advice**).
- Small pliers/tongs for pulling out stones or small objects that tweezers may not be capable of (but never pull a large item out that may have entered a blood vessel – leave this to the vet) from feet or lodged items in mouth/throat where CPR is required.
- Small sterile container for a urine sample.
- Small torch.
- Strips of strong, soft, tape for use as an emergency muzzle.
- Styptic powder or a product to stop small localised bleeds.
- Tube of antiseptic cream.
- Tweezers.

Always check **the use-by date**, if applicable, for any of your First Aid constituents, for example, any made-up liquids such as antiseptics and perhaps the saline solution.

Human medicines

Many over the counter (OTC) medicines that humans use can also help pet dogs and cats. However, do carefully note that because pets are much smaller than humans, the doses will be proportionally much smaller.

It is always best practice to be extremely cautious and check with your vet before giving any human medicines to your pet.

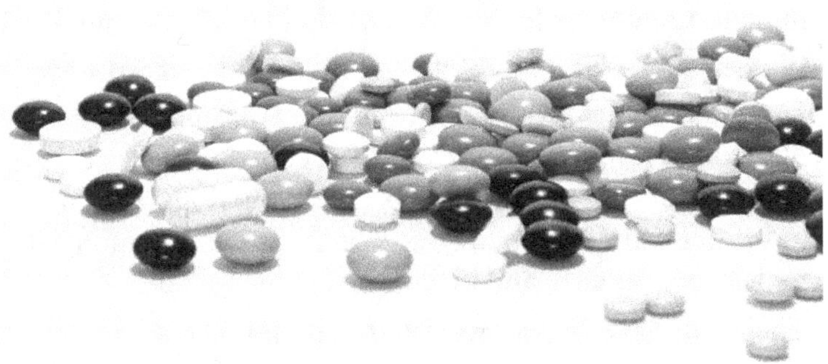

If your pet is on existing prescribed medicines, just like humans, there could be a clash of the interactive ingredients that could cause side effects or even be dangerous. Never try and be a self-made "search-engine vet", as it is your pet's life in your hands.

It's a fact that most people do not tend to have specific pet medicines available at home. Or if they do, there is a good chance they will be completely out of date.

Note that medicines should only be used in those situations between first contacting your vet, under your vet's advice, and waiting for your appointment to see your vet. They must not in any way be used as a substitute for visiting your vet unless your vet expressly indicates their precise use and dose.

While this list is by no means exhaustive, no responsibility can be taken by me in the event of your pet having a reaction to any of the medicines on this list. **Check with your vet before administration** and just have them to hand. Many human medicines contain the same active ingredients as the pet versions, so the temptation is to help comfort and cure your dog or cat by using over the counter products from your own pharmacy or home medicine cupboard. That having been said, you have to remember that human medicines can be, and often indeed are, dangerous to animals.

Human medicines have, after all, been designed with humans in mind. Specific veterinary medicines and medications to treat medical problems in dogs and cats have all been developed over years of research and trials to act very quickly and efficiently.

They will have been developed in many different strengths to cater for the vast array of pet sizes, from Irish Wolfhounds right down to small kittens, thus eliminating the guesswork or numbers necessary to work out just how big – or small – a dose to administer. Human medicines will more often than not also be pet-friendly in taste compared to their human equivalent to help them go down more easily.

> **So, it is always for the best that you consult your vet first.**

We are all very used to buying over the counter preparations at our pharmacy that are usually in liquid, capsule or pill form. You will find these products will usually be categorised by their strength, with pills in milligrams (mg) or micrograms (mcg) and liquids in millilitres (ml) or teaspoon measures.

Some may come with their own graduated mini measuring cup or disposable spoon (which should be washed out with hot water after each use, and also used for the one pet only and then thrown away).

Dogs and cats, as we have already mentioned, because they are much smaller than humans, should never be given the dose recommended for humans on the medicine's packaging. The only exception to this is when either under strict vet instruction/supervision or when it is specific animal medicine from your vet.

The instructions must be followed to the letter.

While pets are animals and have a typical animal digestive system with similar vital organs to those we humans have, their digestive tracts and bodies work a little differently to ours. This means that their breakdown and absorption of drugs can be very different to our own. And, when all is said and done, human drugs have been designed specifically for humans!

WARNING: Medicines for humans, when administered to dogs and cats, will nearly always have an excess of the required constituent active drug because they are designed for humans who, obvious that it may be, are of much larger size than your average pet.

The method for correcting this is to simply work out (using a calculator or good old-fashioned pencil and paper) how much of a 10ml dose for a 60kg human has to be given to a 10kg (or whatever weight) pet.

This is one of the reasons it is so important to know your pet's weight (appreciating it is sometimes difficult to weigh a cat that does not want to be weighed!), not just so you can administer medicines, but so your vet can work out a required dosage over the phone. If you are not too sure, always check with your vet.

Write the weight of your pet in your First Aid kit notebook, clearly remembering to indicate which pet it is, with a description suitable to help a stranger that your pet may not respond to if called by name.

Dealing with dosages and scaling them down

Liquids are very easy to apportion correctly. Take two identical spoons (ensure they are spotlessly clean) and pour out the recommended adult dosage into one of them. Then keep subdividing equally, pouring one of the spoon's contents back into the bottle until you arrive at the dosage you have calculated based on your pet's weight.

Pills can be a little more difficult, especially when you need to cut them down. The easiest method is to grab the pill in the middle using a sterile nail clipper and keep dividing each resultant half until you have the dose you need. If your pet is rather quick on the uptake and refuses pills, despite disguising them in their food, try crushing the pill to powder and sprinkle it in, or on, a treat.

Human medicines that can be used for pets

- Note that while some human medicines will be fine for dogs when used proportionally **(and with extreme care, preferably only with vet advice)** as detailed above, they may not all be safe for cats.
- We have indicated the medicines on our list below that **cannot be administered to cats.**
- The list of potentially pet-safe human medicines below is not exhaustive but just includes some of the more popular OTC human medicines.

A & D ointment

Antibacterial ointment for treating scrapes and wounds. Contains vitamins A and as well as Petrolatum and Lanolin, the two active ingredients that create a protective barrier.

Apply a very thin coating 3-4 times a day for 7-10 days.

Anbesol liquid or gel

An anaesthetic to soothe mouth pain.

Apply with a piece of clean cotton (not cotton wool) once or twice a day for no more than two days. **<u>Only once a day for cats.</u>**

Aveeno Oatmeal medicated bath

Can help soothe itchy skin.

Use as a bath rinse up to three times a week.

Works best when sprinkled under the water being poured into the bath.

Benadryl

Diphenhydramine classed as an antihistamine.

Can alleviate itchy skin, especially when due to insect bites.

1mg is usually dispensed for every half kg in weight of the dog, every 6-8 hours.

Betadine

Povidone-iodine, also known as iodopovidone and marketed as Betadine, is an antiseptic used for skin disinfection and cleansing on or around wounds.

It is usually used full strength to wash the affected area.

Bufferin
A 'buffered Aspirin' (contains antacids to neutralise the acid in the stomach to reduce any potential stomach upset) pain reliever.
Administer around 10-25mg per kg of dog weight two or three times a day.
Must NOT be used on cats.

Burow's solution ("Domeboro" trade name)
A topical antiseptic for minor skin irritation and/or contact with poison.
Applied directly to the wound area on a moistened cotton ball.

Caladryl
A soothing topical lotion for pain and itching.
Apply to the appropriate area.
Cortaid (or generic)
A hydrocortisone steroid anti-itch cream for allergic reactions, eczema, or psoriasis.
Apply once or twice a day as needed.

Dulcolax
For constipation.
A 5-mg tablet once a day or ½ paediatric suppository used once a day.

Epsom salts

A soothing bath soak for irritated, itchy skin.

One cup per nine litres of water, then soak the affected area in the bath.

Iodine

Used as a topical antiseptic.

Provides antimicrobial activity and is effective against bacteria, mycobacteria, fungi, protozoa and viruses and can be used to treat both acute and chronic wounds.

Apply over wound.

Lanacane

Topical anaesthetic forms a protective film over raw inflamed tissue. Its anaesthetic cooling action soothes itching and irritation.

Gauze is used to spread over the infected area.

Must NOT be used on cats.

Maalox Liquid

For digestive upset and excessive flatulence.

Maalox Oral Suspension eases problems of indigestion and related symptoms.

Small dogs up to 7kg – three tablespoons.

Medium dogs from 7kg up to 22kg – four tablespoons.

Large dogs over 22kg – six tablespoons.

Neosporin

For the prevention of wound infection. Apply three to four times daily as required.

Pepto-Bismol liquid

For diarrhoea, nausea, indigestion and vomiting.

½ to 1ml per ½kilo in weight of dog, or ½ to one teaspoon per 2½ kilo up to a maximum of 30ml or two tablespoons up to three times per day.

<u>Must NOT be used on cats.</u>

Preparation H

For a sore anal area.

Apply up to four times a day.

<u>Must NOT be used on cats.</u>

Vicks VapoRub

For congestion.

Rub a small amount on your pet's chin to help with their breathing.

Witch hazel

An astringent/topical antiseptic.

Rub some on the affected area.

It is always a very good idea to consult your vet before administering any of the above human OTC medicines.

A basic summary pet responsiveness chart

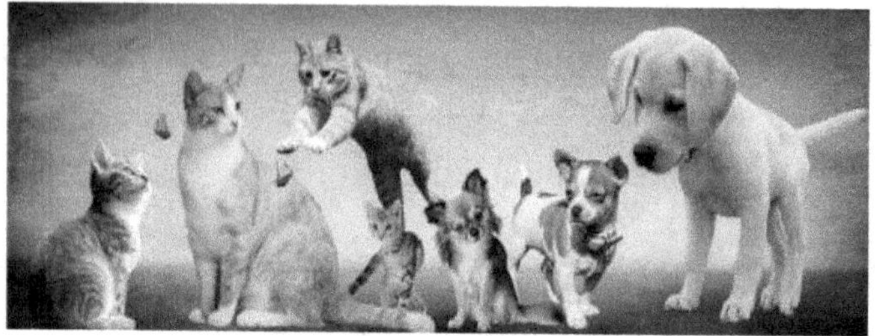

Responsiveness in dogs and cats

NORMAL

Your pet is always alert and responsive to both you and any outside stimuli. If you call him for playtime or a treat he always responds immediately (unless stubborn!)

ABNORMAL

Depressed
Response to sight, smell or touch stimulation is slow
Seems sleepy or reluctant to move

Seen with many illnesses (arthritis, general pain, stomach ache etc)
If no better within 24 hours, call vet

Disorientated, bumps into things
Blank stare
Walks unsteadily, or in circles
Falls to one side

Potential neurological disorder or inner-ear problem
Call vet immediately

SERIOUS

In a stupour
Reponds only when in deep pain

Neuroligical or metabolic problem
Call vet as you take pet to vet hospital

EMERGENCY

Comatose/unable to be woken
Suffers seisures

Severe neurological damage or disruptive injury, toxin or illness
Wrap your pet in a blanket and call vet as you take pet to vet hospital

Perhaps consider making a photocopy and/or take a picture of the chart on your smartphone or tablet and keep it to hand for all human members of the pet's family.

You may care to photograph it and if you have a printer, send it to your PC and print off a copy to keep by your First Aid kit.

A basic health assessment of your pet

Your vet will more than likely only see your pet once or perhaps twice a year, and even then, unless as a result of a medical incident, it may only be for check-ups or the likes of worming. As the owner, you are with your pet every day of the year. This means you in the best position to immediately recognise when things seem not quite what they should be.

For this reason, it is a very good idea to take time out to produce a health-check chart you can refer to for times when you think your pet is off colour.

Remember, except for obvious signs such as, for example, a limp, a cut, or a lump on the body, your pet cannot come up to you and tell you it is feeling under the weather and that it might have a stomach ache. It is up to you to continually keep a look out that your pet does not show any unusual signs of behaviour that may indicate it is not well.

Your pet health-check chart needs to be produced at a time when you know your pet is fit, healthy and very happy with itself. What you need to measure and include on your chart for reference are:

- Capillary refill time
- Colour of skin and gums
- Dehydration test
- Heart rate
- Respiration (breathing) rate
- Responsiveness
- Temperature

You are the one who is most familiar with your pet on a personal level. You should be able to build up a range of health readings that could well be termed as regular.

Once you know what your pet's normality in terms of general health is, you should then be able to identify anything that might seem to be a problem that may need looking into. This knowledge of your pet should assist you with deciding the significance of any condition you might either suspect or even uncover.

This will help you decide what First Aid steps you need to take, as well as make the vital decision whether First Aid will give you time to speak with the vet first, or whether you need to get your pet to the vet immediately.

No acting as an amateur vet please!

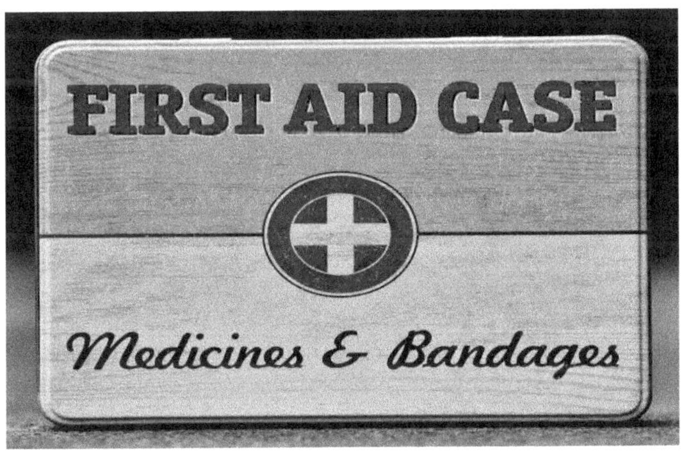

Always remember, First Aid is what it says, that is, it's your first and one-time emergency intervention to help your pet to survive long enough to enable you to get the expert professional medical help needed.

There is no book in the world that can take the place of the vet. It's a false economy, from both a health and monetary point of view, to try and act as and to replace the vet at home.

Pain in pets

It is often quite hard to appreciate when dogs and cats are in pain. The only reliable way you can notice is to be fully aware of their normal behaviour and recognise changes outside that normal behaviour you have come to expect.

Cats - because they tend to be so much more independent and aloof, if they are in pain, they will generally hide away and/or refuse to move.

Dogs - are far more responsive to humans than cats. They will usually be much more open and direct about their feelings at any particular time. They will often hold their paw up, limp and be quite vocal about things, such as whimpering, yelping or even baying.

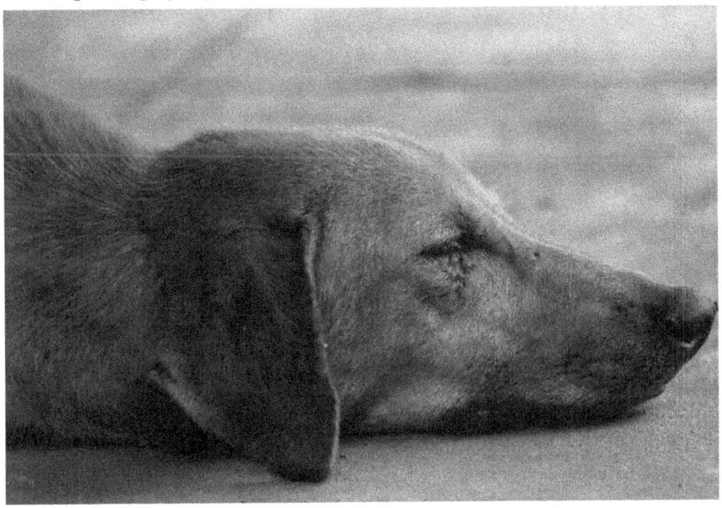

The other signs of hidden pain you may see in pets are behaviours such as refusing to eat or drink and pulling away from you if touched.

They will also seem to have a complete disinterest in everything around them. They may pant, drool, "pull" themselves into a hunched position or hold their head unnaturally. There may be a seepage from the eyes or ears and perhaps ongoing incontinence.

WARNING NOTE - In the case of suspected spine difficulties, fractures or breakages, never use pain relief medicine for your First Aid activities.

While OTC human medicine such as buffered aspirin is often used as a regular pain relief medicine for dogs, it can, and most often will make bleeding worse. Like any medicine, aspirin can be dangerous to give to your pet **(you must never give aspirin to cats)** in First Aid situations when you don't really know what the underlying problem actually is.

This is why you must always leave it to your vet to dispense the safest and most effective pain medicines for your pet following diagnosis.

However, there are nevertheless some safe and effective pain treatments you can utilise during your First Aid application:

- Products such as **Lanacane** that contains **benzocaine**, with their topical anaesthetics, can help numb the pain of for example mouth sores and burns.

Benzocaine should never be used on cats.

- **Hydrocortisone** cream contains steroids that can help with reducing areas of painful inflammation such as minor cuts, scrapes and even insect stings.
- **Ice** can help numb the pain of nearly any skin injury, bruise, or burn within minutes and without being in any way invasive.
- Similarly, a **hot compress** can bring great relief to sore or stiff arthritic joints.

Triage

It's all very well knowing how best to appraise your pet's vital signs and any effects they have on its health. However, you must also be able to very quickly evaluate how severe any problems might be, whether they are medical or physical. This is even more so should there be numerous injuries, say as the result of your pet being run over in traffic.

While it is an absolute necessity to get your pet to the vet immediately, it is advantageous if you do know how to offer emergency First Aid. The big caution here is that, like humans, moving your pet can do irreparable damage if, for example, a broken bone then severs a blood vessel or nerves as a result of being moved. As it is for humans visiting a hospital, this particular procedure is called **triage**. Triage is the process of examining the pet and checking off the problems you determine in order of how serious they are.

Doing this means you can make use of your knowledge of First Aid to prioritise the most serious problems and in essence save your pet's life. Once this is done, you can look at any of the other 'less' serious problems.

There is one thing that people sometimes forget, possibly because they are most probably panicking about their pet, is to check that the immediate surroundings where the incident has occurred are safe enough for First Aid.

It's not much use performing First Aid if you and your pet are not in a safe environment and you are both at risk, such as near a bitten-through electrical flex on a wet floor.

Only when you have assessed the surroundings, should you check your pet and decide what the next 'medical' stage is.

It is universally accepted that where there is a whole-body injury such as shock, or a major internal trauma such as poisoning, these need to take precedence over injuries such as a broken paws or cuts.

Certain injuries, while they may look terrible and will certainly be painful for your pet, if they are not immediately life-threatening, these can be treated after other more serious problems have been attended to.

The first test is the obvious one, namely, does your pet respond to your voice when you talk to it or call it (that is, if they otherwise normally do so when healthy and well – for example, some cats are so independent or haughty that they simply ignore you no matter how much you try to attract their attention). Does the colour of the gums or the time for capillary vessel refill (see after the "list of 10" below) indicate the animal may bc in shock? Are they managing to breathe okay without assistance? An example would be that if a dog has been knocked down in traffic and has suffered a nasty tail injury, this will have to come secondary if your pet has stopped breathing.

The following are the main 10 circumstances identified by triage that must be treated first before attending to any of your pet's other difficulties:

1. Breathing has stopped with no pulse

2. Breathing has stopped but with pulse

3. Unconsciousness

4. Shock, demonstrated by pale gums, breathing that is rapid rather than relaxed, a weak and rapid pulse, skin that is cold to the touch

5. Breathing problems

6. Chest puncture or a large wound
7. Heavy breathing

8. Abdominal puncture or a large wound

9. Total extremes in body temperature, either too cold or too hot

10. Poisoning, stings, ingestion of toxins (and although not so much here in the UK, snakebites).

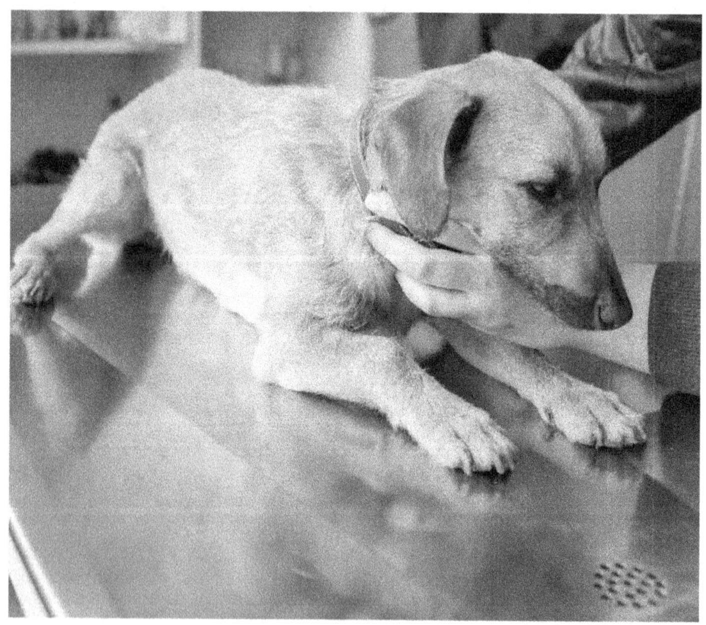

Capillary refill time

Capillary refill test To measure the condition of your pet's circulation, refer to the following chart.		
Capillary Refill Time	**Status**	**Call your vet**
1-2 seconds	Normal	No
2-4 seconds	Moderate to poor; potential dehydration or shock	Yes, as soon as you can
More than 4 seconds	Severe problems; dehydration, shock	Immediately
Less than 1 second	Severe problems; heatstroke, shock	Immediately

Capillaries are those very small blood-containing structures that are located near the surface of the skin. The capillaries, because they are the tiniest and most plentiful form of blood vessel in the body and are so near the surface, are what give this tissue its normal, healthy pink colour. In your pet, they are easiest to see in their gums, just above the teeth. The blood circulation condition of your pet can be investigated by a capillary refill test. You will need a watch or phone that enables you to count in seconds. You need to raise the upper lip of your pet, then gently push your finger against the pink, uncoloured gum tissue. What this does is momentarily push the blood in that spot out of the blood-rich capillaries preventing the normal flow.

If you very quickly then take your finger away, you should see a white, finger-shaped mark left behind for a moment on the gum. Use your watch or phone (a smartphone, if you have one, is best, because you can use the timing feature with your other finger so you can keep your eye on the test) to time how long it takes in seconds for the white spot to disappear and the original pink colour to return. And that's all there is the capillary refill time test!

Colour of skin and gums

Veterinarians generally use the colour of structures such as the "whites" of the eyes and the gums above the animal's teeth to gauge a pet's health. This is because the colour of the skin is normally very hard to see and evaluate because of their coats.

For the gums, if you observe any colour other than normal pink, you need to call the vet straight away or administer First Aid.

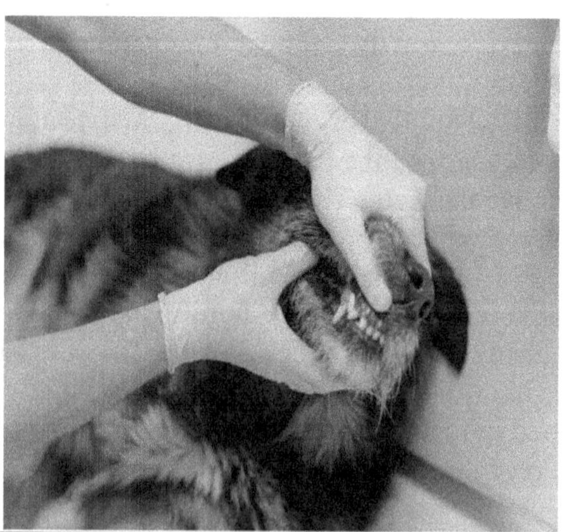

If you see that your pet's gums are black or brown, try and find a pink spot somewhere on the gums (or lips) to evaluate the extent of the disorder. If you can't find a pink spot around the gums or lips, you will need to examine another mucous membrane, such as the vulva or covering over the end of the penis to examine for any pigmentation that simply looks wrong.

Mucous membrane colour test - this quick appraisal chart will help you decide whether your pet needs medical attention.		
Membrane Colour	**Status**	**Call your vet**
Pink	Normal	No
Pale to white	Possible anaemia or shock	Immediately
Blue	Smoke inhalation or suffocation	Immediately
Bright cherry red	Carbon monoxide poisoning	Immediately
Yellow	Liver problems	The same day

Dehydration test

It's surprisingly easy to determine a potential loss of fluid or any dehydration with your pet. The relative elasticity of the skin means that under normal conditions and with balanced water levels, the scruff of the neck is very easy to gently grab hold of. When you pull up the scruff and then let go again, if all is normal, the skin should spring back immediately to its regular position. It's not a bad idea to test the top of the headfirst, because the skin there will probably show the result more easily.

- Where there is only moderate dehydration, the skin will return to normal slowly
- With increased dehydration, it takes the skin longer to return to its normal state
- For very serious cases, where the skin remains pinched up after you've released it, First Aid will be needed immediately to be followed up quickly by veterinary care.

Heart rate

As it is for humans, to measure your pet's heart rate and check whether it is normal or not, they should firstly sit or lie in as relaxed a position as possible. With some pets, this can be difficult, especially with younger ones that may just think you are playing a new game, or others that may not be too happy to either remain still or be handled.

Place the ball of two fingers of your hand (don't use your thumb) on the left side of your pet's body behind the elbow. Identify the feel of the heartbeat and count the number of beats over a 15-second period. You then multiply this beat count by four to arrive at the beats-per-minute rate. To be as accurate as possible, you should repeat this test and count two or three times, and then average your counts out to find a median normal rate.

You also should check your pet's pulse rate as well to become acquainted with exactly how a normal pulse feels. To check this, place your hand on the inside of the rear leg at the point of the mid-thigh near the groin.

Here you should be able to feel the femoral artery pulsing blood through the body near the surface.

Do note that if this is the first time you have tried, you may have some difficulty locating it.

A pulse should be strong, and you should be able to feel it at the same time as each heartbeat.

Where there is injury or an illness, such as heart disease or shock, you will most usually discover a slower-than-normal rate, termed medically as bradycardia.

However, a highly increased heart rate, especially when in the resting position, can also point to shock. Either of these situations will necessitate immediate medical attention. Should the heart stop altogether, your pet will need immediate CPR **and you must have someone contact your vet immediately.**

DO NOT WASTE TIME that could otherwise see you getting to your vet more speedily!

If the pulse is irregular it can point to heart problems. However, a "springing" pulse or otherwise an extremely weak pulse can demonstrate a weak heart output, a drop in blood pressure or shock. All of these will necessitate fast medical attention.

Try to find femoral artery which by placing your finger-tip gently on the inside of the rear leg at the point of the mid-thigh near the groin. You should use your index, middle, and ring fingers to feel for a pulse. It's very strong at this point.

Should you not be able to feel it, and you can't hear a heartbeat by putting your ear to the animal's chest, the heart has probably stopped, and you'll need to initiate CPR.

You should try to identify the femoral artery and pulse points when your pet is alert and well so that you know what you are looking for in the event of an emergency. **You MUST NOT waste time trying to find "things" out about your pet while they are in a critical situation.**

SO BE PREPARED IN ADVANCE.

It also may be somewhat difficult to find the pulse if your pet is in any way dehydrated, depressed, or of course, has low blood pressure.

Remember, unlike humans, pets won't exhibit very strong pulses either in their "wrists", neck or on the front legs.

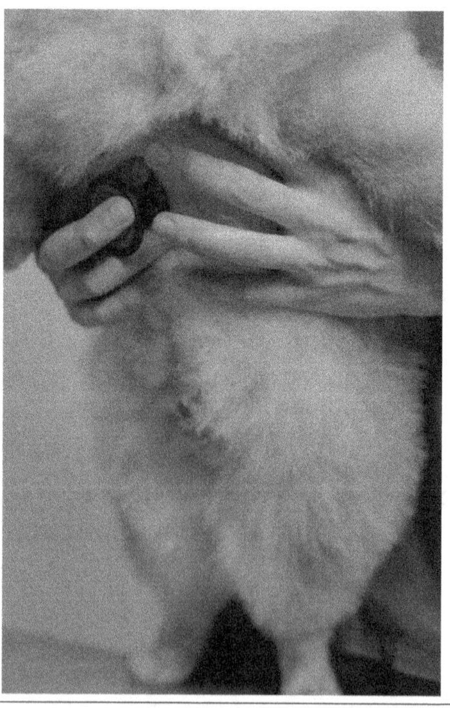

The normal rate for pets. This chart shows the average beats per minute based on your pet's size.	
Pet Normal heart rate	**Beats per minute**
Small dogs (up to 9kg)	70—180
Medium and large dogs (more than 9kg)	60—140
Cats	120-240
Puppies (up to 6 weeks of age)	Up to 220
Kittens (up to 6 weeks of age)	200-300

Respiration

Many people assume that respiration means breathing, which scientifically is not completely accurate.

Respiration is a chemical reaction that technically occurs in every cell in the body. Respiration needs oxygen, and animals obtain their oxygen by breathing.

However, for First Aid, we'll refer to breathing in and out as respiration.

Most dogs will take 10 to 30 breaths per minute, while cats will have a breathing rate of between 10 to 40 a minute.

However, when dogs are hot, or they are exercising, they do breathe much more quickly, and may pant up to 200 breaths a minute, especially if the ambient temperature is much warmer than the normal average temperature.

Cats don't pant to cool off as dogs do, so if you see open-mouthed breathing and panting in cats, these signs are to be considered very hazardous indeed. If you see that your cat is breathing or panting with its mouth open, this is not a normal feline response so you will need to call your vet **straight away.**

Monitoring respiration.

When your pet is resting quietly, anything you hear other than effortless and quiet breathing will call for medical attention and possibly even artificial respiration.

Sign	Status	Call your vet
Effortless breathing, quiet, almost soundless	Normal	No
Respiratory rate Increased	First signs of problems with breathing	Yes. Straight away if it seems that things are getting worse. If increased but not getting any worse, call the vet the same day.
Excessive panting or gasping; dogs exhibit outward-elbow stance; cats sit stooped with head and neck stretched	Emergency. The classic sign of the onset of early respiratory failure	Yes. Straight away
Open-mouthed and/or laboured breathing and showing blue gums.	Emergency. Pulmonary failure; the pet will be suffocating	Yes. Straight away
Very shallow/slow, or breathing stopped altogether with imminent unconsciousness	Emergency. Respiratory failure. Get ready for artificial respiration	Yes. Straight away

Responsiveness

When they are healthy, dogs and cats tend to be both alert and responsive to anything in their surroundings. This all changes when they are ill or have been injured in any way.

- As a result, their behaviour will be somewhat different to the normal behaviour that you expect or indeed are used to.

- The more serious the ailment is, the less response you'll receive from your pet.

- They will appear totally disinterested in what's going on around them.

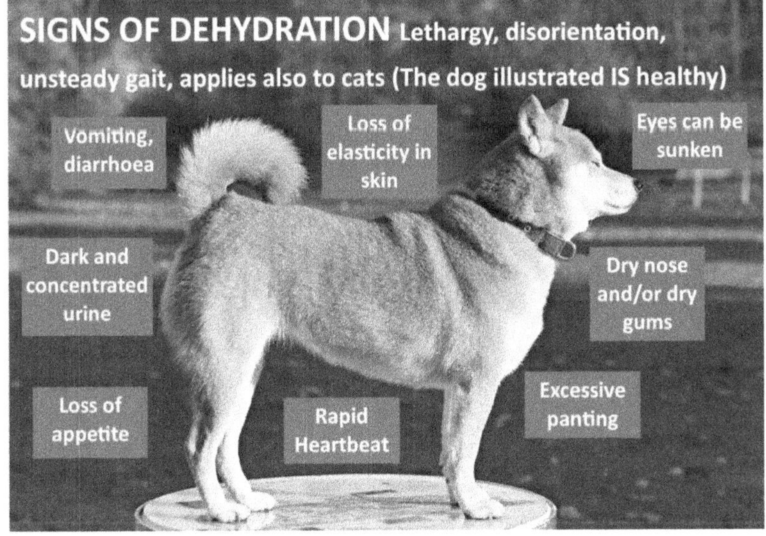

Gauging responsiveness		
Normal, healthy pets are alert, responsive, very curious.		
Consciousness level	**Status**	**Call your vet**
Alert and responsive to both owner and other stimuli; if you call your pet for a treat, they should respond	Normal	No
Depressed; response slow to sight or touch stimulation; may be sleepy or reluctant to move	Common to numerous illnesses	Yes, next day if you can't treat successfully with First Aid
Disorientation; bumping into things, walks very unsteadily, can fall over, walks in circles, stares into space	Potentially neurologic or can be problems within the inner ear	Yes, same day
Stupor; responds only to deep pain stimulation	Neurologic or metabolic problem, serious	Yes, straight away
Either unable to wake or has constant/recurring seizures	Emergency! Severe neurologic damage or possible disruption from disease, injury or poison	Yes, straight away

Temperature

The usual body temperature for dogs and cats is between 37.2° and 39.2° C. Naturally enough, if your pet has just been out to exercise, or has been playing, or running around during summer, it will show an increase of a degree or two, but following a rest, the temperature should return to within the normal range between 37.2° and 39.2° C.

You need to note that a fever may not be hazardous on its own. However, this could indicate a problem that might need First Aid to prevent it worsening to fatal proportions.

Use a rectal thermometer and ensure that you always sterilise it and use it for one pet only. A digital one is best, as there is no glass to shatter or mercury to have to shake down as you need to do when using a traditional bulb thermometer (which needs to be shaken down until it reads 35.5°C).

Coat the measurement probe (or glass bulb end for a traditional thermometer) of a rectal thermometer with either Vaseline, a proprietary mineral oil or K-Y Jelly.

Gently but firmly hold the base of your pet's tail and lift it to access the anal opening. Very carefully insert the probe or thermometer about halfway in. Remember that glass thermometers are much more fragile than digital probes, but on the other hand, if the digital probe is metal it can pierce the tissues. Most modern digital probes should be rounded plastic.

You must keep a firm hold of the tail to restrain your pet and prevent it from sitting down on the thermometer.

Allow about three minutes for a traditional thermometer, or around 40 seconds for a digital thermometer probe to produce a reading. (App-based digital thermometers can produce a reading in around 10 seconds but can suffer from reliability issues). For a traditional thermometer, you need to read the mercury level of it yourself, so remove and wipe clean with a tissue or antibacterial wipe and read the silver column of mercury. (It is always best to follow the manufacturer's precise directions for reading from a digital thermometer).

What is not normal
Depressed and quiet, not very alert, not as quick as expected to respond to noise, touch, smell or stimulation. Sleepy, lethargic.

Very serious
Metabolic or neurological problem. Call vet as on the way to their surgery.

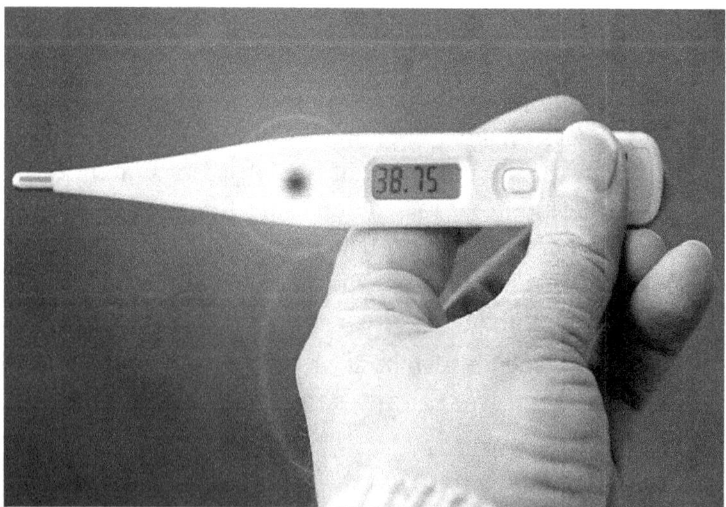

Taking the temperature of your pet
Having taken your pet's temperature, it's very important to know when it's normal or when it signals an emergency.

Temperature reading	Status	Call your vet
41.1°C or higher	Danger, cool your pet down	Immediately
40.5°C	High fever	The same day
40°C	Moderate fever	Yes
39.4°C	Moderate fever	Yes
38.9°C	Normal temperature	No
38.3°C	Normal temperature	No
37.7°C	Normal temperature	No
37.2°C	Normal temperature	No
37.2°C to 35°C	Mild hypothermia	The same day
Under 35°C	Danger, warm your pet up	Immediately

What you need to do
Very common with many afflictions such as stomachache, arthritis, general pain. Call your vet withing 24 hours if there are no visible signs of improvement.

Neurological disorder or something to do with the inner ear.

Call your vet straight away.

An emergency
Severe neurologic damage or possible disruption from disease, injury or poison. Wrap your pet in a familiar blanket and call your vet on the way to their surgery.

Preventing problems

Before we look further into basic First Aid for your pet, it might be worth remembering the updated adage that "*a gram of prevention is worth a kilogramme of cure*". While there is no doubt that you really should be versed in some form of First Aid for your pet, it is no harm in outlining some of the flashpoints that can cause injury or harm.

It is a reality that so many of the emergencies that require the vet's attention could very easily be prevented in the first place. First Aid can without a doubt prove to be a

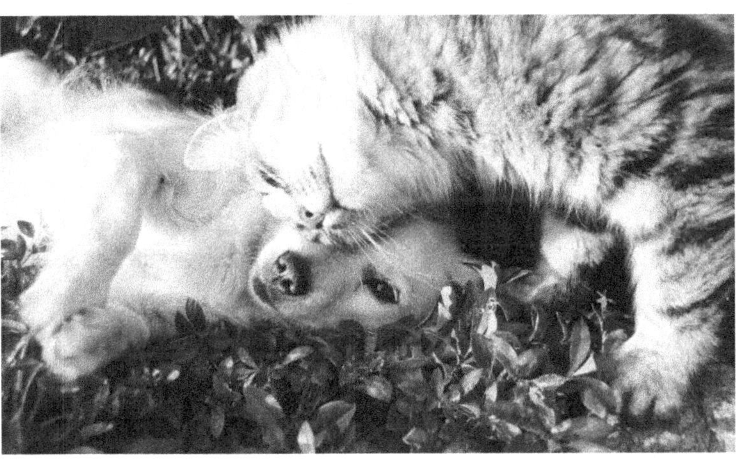

lifesaver for your pet, should something unexpected happens that affects the health and wellbeing of your pet. But a far better way of doing things for your pet is to try and prevent injuries and illnesses in the first place.

And really, it is a shame that in many instances all it would have taken is just a dose of common sense.

Following are some very simple things you can do to help prevent accidents and thus keep your pet safe and sound.

Outside the house

- **Don't allow your pet to run around outside unsupervised**

Despite it now being against the law in the UK to allow your pet to run loose unsupervised outside where you live, it is so incredibly unsafe. You need to keep your pet safe by keeping them inside. There is no reason to ever let pets out unsupervised. Most have no road or path sense.

Yes, cats are fiercely independent, and when they want to go out, they just will. If you have an efficient cat flap and they have been 'trained' how to use it, often, they will indeed use it. Because of their levels of cleanliness and hygiene, they will only go out for a "comfort break" in the back garden, even if you have (which you should) a cat litter tray in your house.

Remember also, when it comes to cats, the old-fashioned idea of "putting them out for the night" is no longer acceptable. They are domesticated, which means they live with you as part of your family, not outside for eight hours at a stretch overnight. Cats generally are quite content to stay indoors most of the time, venturing out only when they need to, and besides, they will also be far safer indoors.

If you allow your pet to wander around outdoors unsupervised, there are several risks to their safety and even to their lives that you are taking.

They can be knocked down in traffic, get into a fight with another dog/cat or even a wild animal, be stolen by an opportunist passer-by, poisoned, shot at with an air rifle, bullied or hurt by a person with no respect for animals, or they can just simply become lost.

You wouldn't let your six-year-old child outside unsupervised, so, do you not think your favourite four-legged member of the family deserves likewise? Your dog will be more than happy just to accompany you on a walk on their lead instead.

Fence them in

If you do allow your pet outdoors unsupervised (and we are not saying that you shouldn't in your back garden), install a strong fence.

It must be tall enough to keep your dog from climbing over it (remember some dogs can grasp and climb with their claws) as well as to keep other animals from climbing in. But do remember that you will rarely if ever be able to completely fence a cat in, because as a rule, they tend to be expert climbers. You can get cat fence barriers, but they can make the garden look unsightly as well as tempt opportunists who, perhaps assuming the barriers are for added home security, think there might be something worthwhile breaking into your house for.

Any fence should be dug well into the ground and also below ground level to prevent your dog from digging its way out and other dogs or animals from digging their way in. And it should be strong enough so that it can't be knocked down by your pet rushing at it and breaking it.

There are other potential consequences leaving your pet outside unsupervised, even in a safe garden. Despite their fierce independence, cats can still fall and fracture bones while climbing.

Any pet can become dehydrated on a hot day if there is insufficient shade for them or if they haven't enough water to drink or they spill their water bowl over. And during winter, the opposite can apply where your pet can so easily get hypothermia from the cold. And bear in mind that when a dog becomes bored through a lack of stimulation, it can become destructive by digging or gnawing where it shouldn't.

Chains, leashes and tethering are out

Like the old-fashioned idea of putting the cat out overnight that we mentioned earlier, similarly, tying a dog with a chain to a post in the garden is similarly no longer an acceptable practice. They have now become far too domesticated to be treated as anything other than a member of the family.

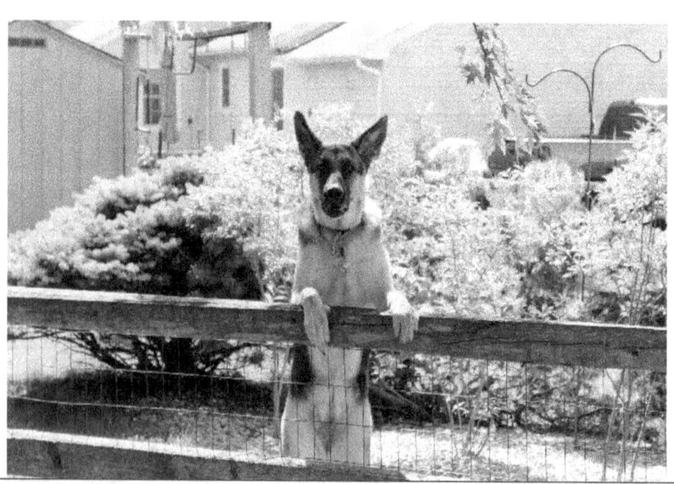

Aside from easily becoming too hot or too cold, a dog can also pick up allergies and viruses, as well as fleas, ticks and other unwanted parasites, not to mention bites from maggots and flies, because a tethered dog is unable to distance itself from its excrement, especially in the heat.

A tethered dog is also not only at risk from choking by winding itself around its tethering post or getting otherwise entangled but can also be at risk from attack by other animals, and sad to say, humans. The dog may, if it becomes excited, cause problems by straining to get at passing animals, cars, bicycles or humans.

Tethered dogs will also suffer from acute boredom and frustration which can lead to destructive behaviour as well as excessive biting, chewing and tearing, which can further manifest itself and continue inside the home.

The ideal outdoor checklist

If you **do** have to leave your pet outside for any length of time, make sure it is happy, safe and healthy. While not exhaustive, the following is a suitable checklist.

- A fully and safely fenced enclosure that provides plenty of room for running, play and exercise
- Somewhere shady to lie down
- A sturdy and comfortable structure to shelter from the weather should it suddenly change before you can bring your pet back indoors
- Several water bowls, filled with water - ensure they can't be broken or easily tipped over by your dog
- Safe and durable toys (that you regularly bring inside and clean)

- Extra flea, tick, and worm protection
- For cats, something to climb on
- Clean up daily from your pet each day

Feed your pet correctly

Feeding your pet on cheap food bulked up with semi-nutritional fillers is no good. Similarly, a diet of human leftovers will not give your pet the nutritional requirements it needs.

All you will end up with is numerous or continuous digestive disorders such as diarrhoea, vomiting and maybe even the development of food allergies. And remember, although they love eating it, chocolate contains a chemical called theobromine, which is poisonous to dogs

Always aim for high-quality pet food, possibly the best you can afford (ask your vet or dog breed association, rather than a potentially unqualified retailer, for advice). As a result, your pet will be healthier from the outset.

Like we humans, the "we are what we eat" rule similarly applies to our four-legged friends. Not only that though, but you will also notice that your pet will need less to feel full if fed on a nutritional and balanced quality diet that it enjoys.

Also, hold back on non-nutritional treats, such as calorie-laden human treat food. All these will do is pile on the weight for your pet, put stress on joints and body, impact mobility and in the long run, shorten your pet's life. And they can potentially cause teeth and gum problems too. They may not suffer from clogged arteries as we humans do, but the unnecessary extra weight will do nothing but help shorten their life.

You can purchase healthy treats instead of those unhealthy ones.

You will be amazed at how much dogs like fruit and vegetable-based treats – apple, green peas, carrot, strawberry, watermelon, banana, broccoli and green beans.

Cats are also known to like very small amounts of cooked carrot, asparagus, green beans and broccoli. And remember that a cat's and dog's basic diet is very different – a dog is omnivorous (manages a variety of food) whereas a cat is very much carnivorous (its evolutionary diet has excluded fruit and vegetables) and cats cannot also perceive sweetness, which means some fruit and vegetables are not at all appealing to eat.

However, don't over face your pets with these treats (no more than 7-9% absolute maximum of their total diet for dogs, even less for cats) and never replace food treats with good old-fashioned affection and playtime. Your pet's best treat is the time you devote to him or her.

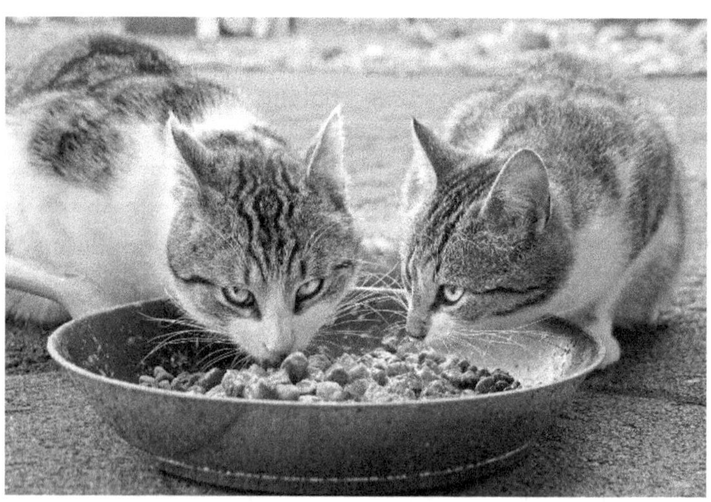

Pets in cars are asking for trouble

This is the most often repeated warning to pet owners.

Never leave your pet in a closed car.

The glass creates a greenhouse effect, even when there is not much sun about, and you will be amazed at how speedily the temperatures inside a car can increase. And the misguided advice that leaving a window open is OK just doesn't work. You'll end up with a stolen car, a stolen pet. . . . or both.

And never tie your pet by their lead outside somewhere you are going. You might find it ends up being "borrowed" by someone without your permission, or if it becomes very uncomfortable due to the weather, it can hurt itself trying to get away.

The best advice is to take your pet along with you into wherever you are going. Or even better still, leave your pet at home if it's a short personal trip out.

Take care you don't accidentally poison your pet

Pets, especially dogs, have a habit of being at their most vulnerable when they spot something that looks like food.

They eat first and suffer the consequences later.

Sometimes it can be a condition called pica (the consumption of non-food substances) and its subdivision coprophagy (the eating of faeces, is one of the most common forms of pica in dogs and cats).

For others such as Labradors, the Romanian Vizsla and sometimes the Weimaraner, they will go out of their way to find and eat what they perceive to be food, as do curious puppies of any breed.

This type of activity can lead to serious blockages in the animal's digestive system as well as poisoning if what they think is food is something like rat bait or maybe a dead small animal that itself died from poisoning.

If you have to use poisoned bait on your property (and you really shouldn't if you keep pets), ensure you keep it and any intended and resultant victims of the poisoning, well out of the reach of your pets.

Other things we humans take for granted that can poison pets are:

Antifreeze: Pets (with the possible exception of cats) find antifreeze has a sweet taste. However, it is extremely toxic and nearly always fatal. The message here is antifreeze should not be left anywhere near where your pet can get hold of it. And if you garage your car at home and it leaks antifreeze, keep your pet out of your garage.

Chocolate: as mentioned previously, chocolate contains theobromine, which is a strong stimulant and is essentially a poison to pets. A large dog may have to eat a large piece to be poisoned, but a small piece can poison a cat or a smaller dog.

Household cleaners: Bleaches, detergent, floor cleaning liquids and toilet cleaners (anything containing either ionic or non-ionic surfactants) can pose an extreme danger to your pet.

If you can do, try to use environmentally friendly alternative products. Make sure you keep the toilet lid down, especially if you have a taller dog or one that is happy to stand on their hind legs and drink out of the toilet bowl.

Insecticides: If you spray chemical insecticides around your house, these can make your pet very ill. Don't spray anywhere near your pet's eating or sleeping area and put feeding bowls away until you've finished spraying and have wiped up. And if you have your home treated for any infestations that require insecticides, it is best you either send your pet to live with another member of the family or a friend for at least a week afterwards.

Lawn and garden treatments: If you use any toxic chemicals or similar products in your garden or on your property, make sure to keep your pet away from them. These can be extremely toxic to them. If you have your lawn sprayed, you will have to keep your pets off it for at least a week.

There are safe organic garden and lawn alternatives, so for your pet's wellbeing, you should perhaps consider using them instead if you can.

Medications: Keep all your medicines, whether for humans or animals, well out of your pet's (and children's!) reach. And don't give your pet a bigger dose, or an "extra bit to be sure" of any medication other than the precise dose recommended by your vet. More is not in any way the slightest bit better, and it could otherwise end up being deadly for your pet. If it says a 5ml dose, administer only a 5ml dose.

Plants: Some houseplants, especially those classed as tropicals (those that grow naturally in a tropical climate) are poisonous (not only to pets but also to humans!). It is suggested you search the internet for those of danger to your pet.

Stimulants: Keep alcohol, tea, coffee, sweets and the likes of lemonade products well out of reach of your pet.

Tobacco: Nicotine is one of the most powerful natural poisons there is, so if you still smoke, keep your cigarette and cigar butts, pipe tobacco, and so forth out of reach of your pet. Also, some of the nicotine replacement liquids for refillable e-cigarette vaping products smell of a quite attractive berry combination, so ensure these are kept out of reach of inquisitive pets, not only because they can poison your pet, but because they can swallow the small e-liquid bottles whole and cause digestive tract problems if they should get stuck.

Neutering your pet

It is a very sad fact that thousands of unwanted and unexpected puppies and kittens are put to sleep every year. Animal shelters around the country can be overflowing with these unfortunate animals who wait for their ill-fated end.

Unless you are a professional and responsible breeder, having your pet neutered or spayed is a very responsible way forward. It can help towards an excess of unwanted puppies as well as help drastically towards the prevention of numerous problems that can otherwise become a threat to health. The likes of disorders in reproduction, unwanted litters, and much-unwanted behaviour can be much more easily managed and prevented.

You'll also eradicate diseases and problems such as those associated with birthing, mastitis, prolapses in the uterine tract as well as some uterine and breast cancers.

As a result, a neutered pet will lead a much lengthier, happy life, and you'll be a proud part of helping to ease the proliferation of unwanted pets.

Making your home more pet-proof and pet safe

Domestic machinery + pets = disaster

You may think an otherwise relatively innocuous and regular activity at home such as using a hairdryer, washing machine or mowing the lawn is harmless. However, your pet will always want to be as close to you as possible and certainly might not always realise that there is a danger present - until it's too late.

Try and keep your pet away from anything mechanical that you use in your home. And it's not much use simply telling your pet to go away.

They may understand your tone, but they won't understand what you are saying and why you are saying it.

If using garden equipment, keep your pet indoors unless you can be 100% sure they will sit somewhere out of harm's way.

Always put sharp objects and miscellaneous items you otherwise take for granted (scissors, screwdrivers, paper staplers, forks) out of harm's way, in the same manner you would do for small children.

Also take care when it comes to cats and their habits of sleeping in warm yet otherwise quite uncomfortable places that we think would be of no interest, such as car engines, tumbler driers and even in an oven that might have been accidentally left open.

Keep doors closed in the first instance and always check inside before operating the equipment again. Always turn off and unplug any electrical equipment when you're not using it.

Does the collar fit?

Often overlooked is the matter of your pet's collar, whether a dog or cat. Owners can accidentally overlook that their pet outgrows their collar whether transitioning from puppy to adult or as an adult animal, putting on a little extra weight that necessitates a bigger collar size. Also, be aware that some collars can have a comfort band on the inside against the fur that can shrink if it gets wet, unsuspectingly reducing the size of the collar.

It is thus important to check your pet's collar regularly to ensure it is a comfortable fit (not too tight **or** not too loose!). The standard test is that you should be able to slip two fingers comfortably between the collar and neck of the animal.

Pet-proof toys

Cats and dogs, especially kittens and puppies, really love to chew things, especially when they are in the process of losing their baby teeth. So, anything that they chew can be swallowed and may end up causing a blockage internally. Objects can also catch in the mouth, throat or jaws and can also break teeth.

Therefore, it is very important not to leave your pet unsupervised at playtime and to be sure that your pet doesn't grab hold of anything it can chew off. And despite it being of a food nature, you must supervise your pet when they chew on bones or dried food 'chew' items.

And don't leave string or similar around that your pet could swallow and tie up their internal organs requiring surgical intervention to correct.

Cords/wires and pets do not mix

A nice length of electrical cord stretched out from an electrical item and under the carpet is very exciting and inviting, especially for the enquiring mind of a puppy or kitten or for a grown-up pet that likes to chew on things.

Sharp animal teeth and any electrical wires never mix.

So never leave kittens, puppies or adult pets who like to chew on their own in rooms where there are wonderful, tasty, electrical cords.

If you do have to leave your pet, make sure all electrical cords are unplugged from the main's socket before you do.

If you can, for a room where you might regularly leave your pet unsupervised, consider running any wires either through a plastic cord protector kit run along the skirting board.

Otherwise, use cord cable nails or a hand cable tacker machine to tack electrical wires or cords to the wall. Both are inexpensive alternatives to losing your pet!

ID your pet

Regardless of whether your pet remains indoors most of the time or not, when not out walking or in the garden with you, you must always have some form of identification on them. A pet can sometimes slip out of your house unnoticed when you open the door to a delivery person, or they may escape from the garden regardless of the precautions you have taken.

And bear in mind that the longer your pet remains lost, the greater chance of them getting injured (and needing First Aid!) or even stolen and passed on.

Aside from a traditional message on a fob attached to any collar, a very good idea is to have your pet microchipped, although this is now a requirement by law for dogs. Also, knowing it has a microchip and if a reward is offered for return, there is a greater chance of your pet being returned home.

Moderation is the way forward

Like people, doing pet things in moderation is the key aspect to ensuring a healthy, happy and long life for your pet.

Aside from plenty of love and attention and plenty of sleep, keeping the food intake to the highest quality, yet at the same time in moderate quantities, together with appropriate levels of exercise will all help towards avoiding you having to undertake otherwise unnecessary First Aid on your pet!

Zoonoses

It is worth mentioning zoonoses (a zoonosis, plural zoonoses, or zoonotic diseases). A zoonosis is an infectious disease caused by a pathogen (an infectious agent, such as a bacterium, virus, parasite or prion) that can be transmitted from an animal (usually a vertebrate) to a human. You should always bear these in mind when coming to the assistance of animals, especially when in an emergency where your concern is solely for the immediate health and wellbeing of the animal that may be unable to help itself. You will find that presenting CPR to an animal in need should not normally cause human illness, but you should always take the utmost care.

The more common transmissible diseases

Ringworm

Ringworm gets its name from the way that a circular area of hair loss and scaling suddenly appears. This appearance usually manifests itself on the ears, face, feet and tail. It can, however, manifest itself with numerous appearances such as large areas with loss of hair/fur, and these can be either with or without seeping or crusts, and may or may not be of irritation to the animal. Ringworm is also known to cause infection to both toenails and the beds of nails.

Unfortunately, it is not always possible to directly attribute the manifestations above as being caused by ringworm, so you can't go on just what you observe.

However, if you do suspect ringworm, make sure you wear appropriate protection such as PPE gloves, gowns and masks and make sure you change these items of PPE between different animals you may handle.

Rabies

You don't need to be reminded how dangerous rabies is, as it is something that should be at the back of every pet owner's mind. Rabies is a viral disease that causes inflammation of the brain in mammals and human. Early symptoms can include fever and tingling at the place of exposure, accompanied by central nervous system disturbance.

What you will notice are very severe changes in normal behaviour coupled with unexpected paralysis both of which will get worse as time passes. Sometimes you will notice varying degrees of change in regular behaviour which may include degrees of apprehension, hyperexcitement, irritation and nervousness together with a very sudden loss of appetite and total lack of interest in food.

They can also become quite aggressive, and you may see a wild animal with rabies suddenly stop being fearful of humans or nocturnal animals suddenly out and about during the day.

Other aspects can see an otherwise unsociable or unfriendly (towards strangers) pet suddenly wanting to be friends with everyone, or a very social pet wanting to be left completely alone.

Scabies

Scabies is a very contagious disease affecting dogs. The mites which cause this extremely irritating disease do tend to be very specific to one host, but any animals or humans coming into contact with an infested dog or cat may well also become infected. The infestation manifests itself as a severe itch with crusts and scabs on the chest, ears, elbows and feet.

The basics

Some initial First Aid techniques to make yourself aware of.

Owners of pets are used to dealing with those everyday complications such as upset stomachs and diarrhoea, small cuts in the fur, eye and ear infections. And they usually know what they have to do until faced with the situation and panic sets in despite all the latent knowledge.

A knowledge of First Aid and how to apply it is not only beneficial but can be a lifesaver for your pet. It is appreciated that it is human nature to look at pet First Aid as being only for those 'real' emergencies, such as electric shock by chewing through an electric flex or being knocked down by a cyclist. However, by and large, most pet owners will rarely, if ever, come face to face with a full-blown pet emergency, or for that matter, an equivalent human emergency. But it can happen.

Basic First Aid techniques can be useful for many, many dog and cat conditions. This can be anything from a cat cold to a rose thorn that needs removing from your pet's paw, to a broken paw or a wasp sting. But what you mustn't underestimate is that under certain traumatic circumstances for your pet, First Aid can save their life.

Restraining your pet safely and humanely
While First Aid is a natural responsive 'act' that humans are familiar with for saving lives and safeguarding their health, animals don't understand this when they are unwell.

Certainly, if awake at the time, the intervention of a human suddenly attempting to do something they are so unfamiliar with, namely, First Aid will be strange to them. As a result, you certainly will not be able to anticipate your pet's reaction to your attempts. So, you need to have some form of humanely kind restraint should you have to curb your pet's movements and activities.

A restraint serves three primary and important features:

- It prevents you from being either bitten or clawed by your injured pet when you are providing First Aid
- It prevents your pet from making their injuries any worse
- It helps keep your pet in one place to enable wound examination and First Aid treatment.

Some methods of restraining

There are various restraint methods, each of which works well for particular injuries. One of the basic choices you must make is to ensure you pick a method that allows you full access to the specific injured area.

What you do need is two people, one to hold and restrain the pet while the second carries out the necessary First Aid. It is an important factor that you are in a comfortable position to be able to administer the help needed, because if you are, say, hunched uncomfortably over your pet while trying to apply treatment, this makes it all the more difficult a task for you.

Smaller pet: you need to place them on a tabletop so that they are at convenient waist level for treatment.

Medium size to large pets: best treated on the floor where you can kneel beside them and also, an injured larger pet will be very difficult for one or two people to lift and avoid further injury to

Dogs with prominent eyes, such as Pugs and Pekinese: Do not hold these breeds of dogs around the neck, as any undue pressure can pop their eyes out of their sockets.

The reclining restraint - What you need to do is to place your pet on their side, ensuring the injured area is facing upwards. With one hand, firmly but gently take hold of the ankle of the foreleg that's against the ground while pressing your forearm gently across your pet's shoulders. Using your other hand, take hold of the ankle of the rear leg that's laying directly on the ground while pressing that same forearm across the dog's hips.

This particular method is great for medium size to large dogs and it is also one to use for dogs that have prominent eyes, for example, Pugs.

The stretch restraint - This is suitable for cats and smaller dogs. Gently take hold of your pet with one hand by the loose skin at the back of the neck, which is called the scruff. Hold both rear legs with your other hand. Now, you need to gently and carefully stretch your pet out by holding them against the table or worktop. Consider wearing a glove on the hand you use to hold your pet's feet.

The hugging restraint - With this method, you should bring one arm under and around your dog's neck, as if you were attempting a wrestling half-nelson. You hold him to your chest with one arm while with the other, grasp gently but firmly under and around his chest and pull him closer against your body. This method is most suited for those dogs that weigh more than nine kilos. It is an especially practical method when trying to keep the abdomen, legs, chest, and back still.

The kneeling restraint

As we have already mentioned, if you put pressure on the neck of dogs with prominent eyes, such as Pugs or Pekingese, this can cause their eyeballs to pop out. So, you cannot hold these breeds with a neck grip or by the scruff of their neck should they need First Aid. You must place your dog on the floor between your knees facing away from you. You then gently put one hand on top of your dog's head with the hand under or around his jaws to steady the head, while another person treats the area. This is also a good method to give pills to cats.

How to make an Elizabethan (lampshade) collar

We've all seen pets at one stage or another wearing what we term as a 'lampshade' collar restraint, which is otherwise technically referred to as an Elizabethan collar, named after the giant ruff seen around the neck of an Elizabethan lord of old. These can be purchased in a variety of sizes to fit any pet, and their main function is to stop dogs and cats from reaching any injuries with their teeth. The collars also stop pets from clawing at any facial sores or injuries they may have.

You can generally purchase them from pet stores, from your vet or online. You can also make one yourself if you need to, but by and large, they are very inexpensive, so buying one makes it much easier and means you are always prepared.

If you do need to make one yourself, you need to measure your pet's neck and the distance from the tip of the nose to the collar. Mark out these measurements on a piece of rigid cardboard or preferably plastic. Then you make a V-shaped cut from the outer edge to the inner circle. Use a pointed object such as a hobby or wood makers awl, or even a knitting needle, to punch holes along and through both edges of the collar. Then thread some yarn or a long shoelace through the holes to keep the collar in place around your pet's neck.

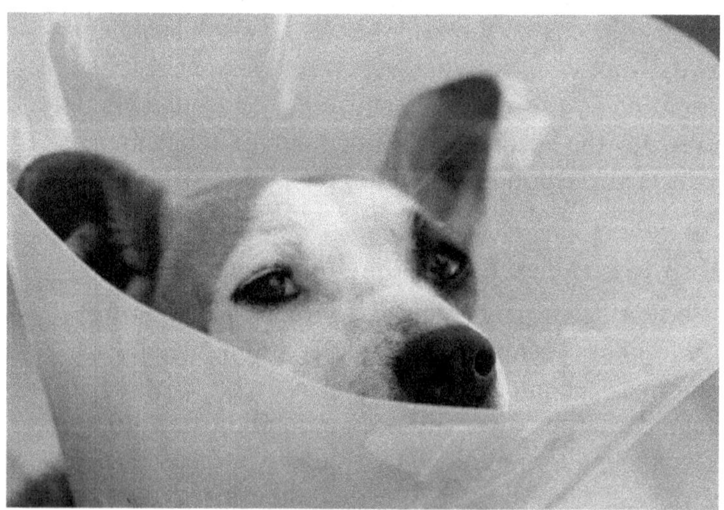

Muzzles

You will find that even if your pet is a gentle giant that would normally not even say 'boo' to a goose, they can simply reflex bite (or scratch) if they have been hurt and are in pain when you examine them.

If your pet is not used to, or has otherwise never needed a muzzle, while you can always purchase one from pet stores if you haven't one to hand, you can very easily make one. This can be difficult for brachycephalic dogs such as bulldogs and pugs as well as for cats, because they haven't the nose and snout to tie closed with your homemade muzzle.

An acknowledged way around this is to use a pillowcase. Gently place it over your pet's head and hold it around their neck (assuming you don't need to access the head area!). You will find that your pet may stop struggling simply because they can't see what's now going on. And if you find your pet has been overheating, you can dampen parts of the pillowcase (do not be over-enthusiastic with your dampening, as you do not want to cause your pet breathing difficulties) to provide a temporary form of cold-water wrapping.

Naturally enough, if your pet is a long-nosed breed, it will be much easier to place a muzzle on. You can use a variety of cloth materials to make your muzzle, providing they are suitable in length and don't have anything on them that could pose a danger to your pet, such as a zip end, button or chemical residue.

Some temporary muzzle materials:

- Spare leash (if made from soft material)
- Denier stockings
- Gents' tie

- Long bandage

Very carefully loop the material you have chosen around your pet's jaw and gently but firmly tie it in a single knot (half hitch) on the top of the nose. Then, bring the ends of what you have tied back down under the jaw and tie another single knot. Finally, pull the ends behind the base of his neck and tie them in a bow or knot behind the ears. This muzzle you have made should hold the jaws closed so your pet can't bite or nip. Don't forget to praise and make a fuss of your pet as you complete each phase of the homemade muzzle.

Artificial respiration and CPR (cardiopulmonary resuscitation)

Introduction

As it is for humans and virtually all other mammals, your pet's cardiopulmonary system keeps going and never stops – unless interrupted by illness or death. The lungs provide oxygen for the blood to carry around, while the heart moves that blood around the body. Once the blood has done a full trip around the body and returns to the lungs once again, the oxygen has been taken out and used where it's required, so that the blood can take on a fresh oxygen supply from the lungs once again and repeat the process.

It follows that anything interrupting your pet's breathing or heartbeat and starves the brain of oxygen, as would be the similarly case for humans, will simply cause a loss of consciousness and potentially - and very speedily - complete irreversible brain damage. So, you must act fast. And if you have never done so before, it can be somewhat daunting. It really is like the way you see it done to humans in television medical dramas. Just don't panic.

Artificial respiration

When having breathing or circulatory difficulty, you will find that pets will usually enter respiratory arrest first. What will happen is that while the breathing ceases, the heart may continue to beat for a short while afterwards.

Therefore, you must begin artificial respiration straight away if you want (which of course you will) to save your pet's life.

It is very easy to say, but you must stay calm.

Therefore, it is so important to have someone else available to drive. You can work on keeping your pet alive while they drive. You will often find that a dog or cat can still be saved by their owner breathing for them even after as long as an ½hour or more.

If your pet is very cold, it may be that they breathe much more slowly than usual. Therefore, it is very important to be sure that the breathing has stopped. The first visible signs are to check whether there is a rise and fall of the chest. The secondary check for breathing is to hold your hand to your pet's nose. If indeed your pet is not breathing, quickly check their mouth as the gums will turn blue from lack of oxygen. However, you must be very quick and methodical about this.

You also must check to see if your pet's airway is clear before you start artificial respiration, as all your efforts will be otherwise wasted if you can't get oxygen down into your pet's lungs. You can quickly check this by opening your pet's mouth and looking inside for any foreign object (to save time perhaps do this at the same time you check gum colour - this is why it is helpful to have a small pocket torch in your First Aid kit).

If you detect that your pet's airway is in any way blocked, if you can, grab the tongue and pull it outward to dislodge the object.

If you must, reach in with your fingers, or otherwise carefully with small pliers or tongs to grab it.

However, if you can't manage to get hold of it, use the Heimlich Manoeuvre as follows below to dislodge an airway blockage.

The Heimlich manoeuvre

Abdominal thrust, also known as the Heimlich manoeuvre, is a basic First Aid procedure used to treat upper airway obstructions by foreign objects. The American doctor Henry Heimlich is often credited with its discovery.

Pets, like young children, will put all kinds of things in their mouths. And if one of those 'all kinds of things' go down the wrong way, it can quickly obstruct the airway and breathing. When this happens, performing the Heimlich manoeuvre will most certainly help towards potentially saving your pet's life.

- **It can be a very useful exercise to try out the Heimlich manoeuvre on a stuffed toy of approximately the same size as your pet. This will give you some idea of what will be required of you to perform it, as well as the relative size of your own hands and body in relation to your pet. It really is not like grabbing a human around the chest.**

If necessary, perform the manoeuvre two or three times in succession. Then check to see if you have managed to dislodge any otherwise stuck object. If you find you haven't managed, continue the manoeuvre in your car while someone drives you to the vet.

Just be mindful that if you have ever performed the manoeuvre on a fellow human, you will never need to use as much pressure on your pet, and while the theory remains the same, the practice is somewhat different.

For a cat or small dog

Hold your pet's back against your stomach with their head up and feet dangling down. Place your fist just underneath the rib cage. You will be able to feel this soft, hollow place easily. Push inwards toward your belly and upward toward your chin, both at the same time. Use a strong thrusting action to help dislodge the object.

For the larger dog

If you own a larger dog who gets into breathing difficulty through a blocked airway by swallowing something they shouldn't, lay them down on the floor on their side and kneel behind with your knees into their back and head pointing towards the left. Lean over the dog and place your fist just below the rib cage pressing very abruptly inward and upwards towards the head.

Once you have succeeded in opening the airway, you can then begin your rescue breathing regime.

1. For a large pet, lay them on their side (it will be easier to support a smaller pet in your lap) and straighten the neck by lifting the chin so that the throat then provides a straight route into the lungs.

2. You won't be able to achieve full mouth-to-mouth resuscitation because, unlike humans, you won't be able to seal your pet's lips with your own mouth. As a result, too much air can escape. What you need to do is close your pet's mouth with one or both hands to seal it.

3. You now have to place your mouth wholly over your pet's nose (with the smaller pet, your mouth will cover both his nose and mouth) and then blow with two quick breaths, watching to see if the lungs expand. You will find that the air will go straight through the nose and into the lungs if you have the mouth fully and correctly sealed.

4. You want to blow air in just firmly enough to move your pet's sides. You will find that with a very large dog, this will take some blowing effort. Do remember to only blow gently for cats and tiny dogs, as you could very easily rupture their lungs. Between each breath, do allow air to naturally seep from the lungs before giving the next breath. Give around 15 to 20 breaths per minute until your pet begins breathing on their own, or you arrive at the vet's.

Should you need to give your pet artificial respiration, hold their mouth shut with one hand around the muzzle, cover their nose with your mouth and blow gently into the nose until you see the dog's chest rise.

Cardiopulmonary Resuscitation (CPR)

CPR combines artificial respiration with external heart compressions. This assists with moving blood around the body should the heart stop beating. Follow the instructions for rescue breathing and alternate this with standard chest compressions. Two people should perform CPR, with one doing the breathing for the pet while the other person undertakes the chest compressions.
To assess whether your pet's heart has stopped, what you need to do is place the palm of your hand flat against the dog's lower chest area straight behind the front left elbow. Here you will be able to feel for the heartbeat. You can, providing you are in quiet enough surroundings, also place your ear against the identical spot and listen.

You can also try feeling for the dog's pulse in the femoral artery. This is the vessel located adjacent to the surface at the groin on the inside of the thigh. What you need to do is place three fingers flat against this area and press gently, but firmly, and you should be able to feel it. Do note that pets that have stopped hearts won't respond to anything at all. A touch test you can do is to squeeze your pet firmly between the toes or gently tap the eyelid. If the dog doesn't blink or flinch, you need to commence CPR immediately.
Should you need to provide CPR to a medium-size or large dog, you need to first lay them on their side on a hard surface (such as the floor to save trying to lift and further damage your pet or hurt your own back) and place a small pillow under the lower part of the dog's chest. Then place one hand near the highest point of the chest wall and place the other hand over the first and use both hands to compress your dog's chest.

Be firm but careful, just in case there are other underlying causes you may further exacerbate that may have originally stopped your pet breathing and their heart beating. But do bear in mind that your primary task is to get your pet's blood circulating and lungs breathing.

For cats and small dogs that weigh less than nine kilos

The *"cardiac pump technique"* is one where compressions are carried out straight over the heart to essentially squeeze it and start it pumping blood again. This technique is suitable for all cats and dogs that weigh in at less than nine kilos. You will first need to place your pet on their side on a comparatively flat, firm surface.

To competently carry out this technique, you need to locate the centre of the heart, which you will find where the elbow point of your pet crosses their chest. You will need to carefully bend your pet's front left front leg backwards to do this

Cup your hand over your pet's chest at the point just behind the elbows. You will need to squeeze quite firmly, pressing in just over a centimetre deep with your thumb on one side and your fingers on the other.
When it comes to puppies and kittens, because of their size relative to the human hand, you should be able to perform the compressions between your fingers. You do this by supporting your pet in the palm of your hand, and with your thumb over the heart and your fingers on the other side gently squeeze rhythmically to make the heart pump.

Vets recommend a rate of around 80 to 100 compressions a minute which is just a little over one per second.

This can be quite difficult if you have never done this before. If you can get to between 60 and 100 compressions per minute, you're doing extremely well.

For medium and large dogs weighing more than nine kilos

Dogs that weigh in at more than nine kilos generally have very strong bones and plenty of space between their ribs. This means that compressions won't affect their hearts.

 For this reason, vets suggest that as an alternative to pumping above the heart, you use the *"thoracic pump method"*. This is where compressions are carried out at the highest part of the chest.

What is being done using this method is the pressure within the chest cavity changes quite dramatically with the resultant increasing and decreasing pressure moving the blood onwards.

You do this by putting one hand on top of the other against the dog's chest and push down 25% to 50%.

For a barrel-chested dog

If your dog is a breed such as a bulldog with quite a barrel-shaped chest, then you will need to place the dog flat on its back. Kneel, cross the paws over the breastbone and place the abdomen between your legs. Holding onto the dog's paws, undertake the chest compressions by pushing downward directly over the breastbone.

If you find that your dog moves around somewhat while you are undertaking the chest compressions you are best placing the dog on its side and continuing as above. You should aim to alternate between breaths and compressions, with one breath given for every five compressions for any size pet.

Continue the CPR until either your pet regains consciousness, or you reach the vets.

Acupuncture Resuscitation

Acupuncture used in Chinese medicine on both people and animals has been around for over 2,000 years. Many vets think that there is one single acupuncture point, that in the centre of the narrow slit that occurs in the upper lip, which could resuscitate your pet.

This is because stimulating this point releases epinephrine, a natural occurring adrenaline, which is otherwise a drug that is used for cardiac arrest, to stimulate the heart and breathing.

Do note that acupuncture should never replace CPR. However, it is worth a try where a series of sharp jabs to this point with a clean needle, pin, or even your sharp fingernail could otherwise revive your pet should your CPR fail. You must be able to efficiently and accurately insert the needle down to the bone and wiggle it back and forth.

CPR in summary

In summary, when examining your pet to see if CPR is necessary, do your "**ABC**"

A - AIRWAY - is the airway open?

B - BREATHING - is your pet breathing on its own?

C - CIRCULATION - can you detect a heartbeat and a pulse?

Your mini survey needs to include a check on:
1. Mucous membrane colour
2. Refill time for capillaries
3. Evidence of bleeding
4. Level of consciousness

While there is the need for speed with CPR, appreciating your pet is one of the family and you want to do whatever you can to save their life, try not to panic and be as calm and methodical as you can. Also, be systematic and don't change your methodology because you may think because there is no immediate or visible response you are not doing what you need to. Provided you follow the steps above, you **will** be doing what is necessary and all you can.

CPR will not always be successful. Even highly trained and experienced vets sometimes cannot "restart" a pet's body. If any attempt you make to undertake CPR does not work on your pet, please know in your mind that you did everything you could to save your pet's life.

How to clean wounds

When an animal's skin is torn or broken, bacteria or other foreign matter, and this may also include the animal's fur itself, can easily contaminate any wound present and potentially cause infection. And despite what many people say, a dog's tongue, when it licks a wound, does not provide any anaesthetic or disinfecting properties whatsoever – just think what and where a dog can lick during one day!

Bleeding is, despite looking very disconcerting at the time it happens, a normal body cleaning mechanism to help flush hazardous material out from the bloodstream/body. Never cleanse wounds that are bleeding excessively, as this will just prolong the bleeding or even make it increase in volume through disturbing the clotting and natural healing process.

However, if you detect a wound that isn't bleeding, the cleaning you do as part of your First Aid treatment will go a long way to help your pet and keep it a great deal safer in the initial short term.

Any long fur your pet has that might invade the wound or gets in the way has to be very carefully cut away to keep it both out of or sticking to, the injury. If you're using scissors to cut the fur it's a good idea to first slide both your index and second fingers through the fur and hold them against the wound. Cut the fur level with your fingers, leaving approximately a 2½cm border around the wound. Any wound on your pet's body will invariably be sore and uncomfortable for them. You'll find that even the most moderate of touches will be painful should the skin be broken.

What you need to do is very gently paint on some water-soluble lubricant such as Vaseline with a brand-new cotton bud (ensuring none of the cottons on the bud sticks to the would area). The cut fur will then stick to the Vaseline but will wash out very easily when required. By far the best and most reliable way to clean a wound is to flush it well with cool water or sterile saline solution (check if using contact lens saline – some are not just saline and can sting wounds) to wash out any foreign particles. Ensure the stream of water is not too harsh that it hurts your pet.

You can then follow your initial cleansing with a non-stinging antiseptic solution to disinfect the wound – the best method is to dilute your chosen antiseptic with distilled water and to the colour of straw. You can then decant it into a plant sprayer. You are best using a brand-new sprayer that has itself been thoroughly washed out followed by a good number of squirts of the solution through it that you intend to use prior to application on your pet. Spray the injured area completely. Once you are happy that you have fully disinfected the wound, very gently dab it dry with sterilised gauze pads or a clean, lint-free/particle-free cloth.

Bandaging techniques

There is no doubt that some injuries will heal better when allowed the magic of natural uncovered air healing. Meanwhile, other injuries will most certainly heal more efficiently when bandages are used briefly as part of your emergency First Aid activities. But do be mindful that for first aid, a bandage is more than often used only temporarily until you can get the correct treatment from your vet or animal hospital.

Bandages will help to:

- Control any bleeding with the mild pressure they exert
- Prevent your pet from chewing at, scratching or licking their injury
- Keep any wounds clean and dry
- Protect the wound from further airborne infection
- Absorb any leakage from the wound
- Encourage healing

If you do put a bandage on your pet, you have to ensure that initially it is changed daily (unless it gets wet during the course of the day, when it must be changed immediately – you will need to ensure it stays dry) and then once the wound begins to heal that it is replaced every day or two. Should there be any swelling seen either above or below the bandage, this usually indicates that it's wrapped too firmly. If you see that your pet might be chewing at or licking the bandage, or that there's a particularly bad odour coming from it, you should remove the bandage instantly and check that there's not an infection or something equally as sinister occurring.

A homemade bandage

It is only honest to say that individually packaged, commercially manufactured sterile pads will always be best for your First Aid kit. However, if you haven't a commercially-produced bandage to hand (but remember, in an emergency, you won't have time to hang around making homemade bandages!) and should you make your own bandage, it needs to contain a quality absorbent pad, gauze, and bandage tape, and should be prepared well in advance of an unexpected emergency and be placed in their own sterile bag in your pet First Aid kit.

The absorbent pad

Paper towels and other paper products which are without a doubt absorbent and relatively sterile, have the habit of sticking to wounds and tend to be difficult to remove later when the wound dries. Any absorbent material that's 100% clean and is particle and lint-free is usually fine for First Aid. If you only have paper-based products available, smear some Vaseline or other medical lubricant product the wound before bandaging. These products make it easier easy to wash away any remaining 'stuck' paper later.

Gauze

A generous length of gauze from a roll is the best to use to wrap around the pad to keep it in place. Don't wrap it around too tightly, as injuries can often become swollen if they either get worse before they get better, or similarly, start to swell as they heal. Should this occur, it can not only interfere with blood circulation but also be very uncomfortable for your pet.

As a form of 'insurance', always do the two-finger test when bandages are wrapped in place around your pet, that is, ensure you can comfortably get two fingers under the bandage you have tied. A very good rule of thumb is to keep binding the gauze by approximately a third of its width each time you wrap.

You can use other materials from around the home if you don't have gauze to hand (but you should always by default have a roll of gauze in your pet First Aid kit). Any other material with a little bit of elasticity should do the trick, such as perhaps a length of an old pair of tights, the material from an old t-shirt or similar will suffice as a temporary wrap-around bandage. Just ensure it is clean and not either rough or fluffy.

The tape

Without a doubt, medical quality Elastoplast is the best to use to secure a wound bandage, and, you should always have a roll in your First Aid kit. But if you don't, most adhesive tapes will do the job, although packaging 'sticky' tape can be quite 'hard' and not very malleable for sticking around a pet's limb.

If you have to improvise, make use of your pet's fur to bind the bandage to it so that it stays in place when applied.

If you don't have any sticky tape to hand, you can temporarily use strips of plastic food wrap which will adhere to itself when wrapped around a bandage. But use it on a strictly temporary basis only as the wound won't be able to breathe and heal. And, of course, once again, the two-finger rule applies again here.

Special methods you can use for bandaging

There are numerous ways you can apply a bandage to the various parts of your pet's body. Do be mindful that while you want to be as effective as you can, there is no substitute for veterinary intervention to ensure the health and well-being of your pet following an accident or unexpected medical incidence. Always clean and disinfect any wounds as best as you can before applying your bandages.

Legs, paws and pads

Firstly, start by making sure the injury has been completely cleaned, then disinfected and finally dried off, taking extra care not to start the bleeding again if you have already stemmed any bleeding that was originally present. Place a gauze pad (or equivalent as we discussed in the previous section) under your pet's wounded paw. Cut a double length of gauze roll (or your substitute) and roll it out on the paw, working your way from the front of the animal's foot, up over the toes and then under the paw. Using just a single ply wrapping of the gauze roll around the paw, begin your wrapping at the toes and carefully move up until you cover the piece of gauze you originally folded underneath. Make sure to use an even binding pressure and slightly overlap each successive layer over the previous layer.

While it is certainly not an easy task, you must try to keep any bandages you apply as dry as you can. As the paw pads of animals are very prone to sweating, you have to allow the gauze to breathe, which is why the temporary fix of using food-quality cling-film is not the most appropriate, as it keeps the moisture in.

Ideally, apply the adhesive tape to the very top edge only of any bandage you put on the paw. You can always finish by putting a cotton athletic sock on the paw to help protect and preserve the bandage. Do cut it to fit and then use some adhesive tape to attach it to your pet's fur. This will also stop your pet from gnawing or licking at the wound.

Tail

If a part of your pet's tail is injured, you need to place a pad on the area affected and tie it with some gauze or with some strips of your gauze replacement. Then you need to place a cotton tube sock over the end of the tail to cover the pad you have affixed and to cover at least up to two-thirds of the length of the tail.

Then, beginning near the tip of the tail, criss-cross your adhesive tape over the sock, beginning towards your pet's body. Take the tape at least 5cm further than the end of the sock onto your pet's fur. Then do the same diagonal binding with your tape in reverse from the body of your pet down to the tip of the tail. This application makes it difficult for your pet to pull the bandaging off. Again, this is suitable only for First Aid applications and you must seek veterinary advice for anything other than a minor tail abrasion.

Ears

Should there be any injuries sustained to your pet's ears, the best advice is to apply a bandage to the entire head. It is very difficult to bandage just one ear.

The most efficient method is to fold your pet's ears over their head (assuming it is not a serious injury needing immediate medical attention) using a gauze pad or adhesive bandage, making sure to cover the injured part. Join the ends of your bandage to one another with tape. Roll some gauze around the head, covering the ears and then gently but firmly under your pet's throat so that the folded ears stay in place.

If you haven't any gauze any clean, flexible material will do, such as the sleeve from a cotton shirt or T-shirt or even a sock that you have cut the toes from. Whatever you do use can be taped to your pet's fur so it is held in place. You may have to think about using an Elizabethan Collar (or lampshade as it is sometimes referred to) that we referred to earlier.

Neck

For minor neck injuries, place an absorbent pad over the wound and use a gauze roll to hold it in place. To keep it in place, do multiple wrapping, but not too tightly, making sure that breathing is not restricted if your pet can lie down.

Chest and shoulders

Again, for any wounds to the chest or shoulder, place an absorbent pad over the wound. You want to wrap it using a figure of eight pattern over the pad, alternating back over the top of the pad itself, in front of the forelegs and around the chest of the animal. Any tape or gauze used to tie the bandage in place should finish at a point where your pet can't gnaw or pull it off.

Hips and flanks

Use the same figure of eight approach for injuries to the chest or shoulders as above, this time alternating around the stomach and in front of and between or behind the rear legs. You can also use an item of clean male boxer shorts underwear to protect any wound in this area. Pull it up over the hind legs, let the tail stick out of the fly area and use an adhesive bandage or tape to fix it to your pet's stomach area.

Bandages for the body

If your pet injures its stomach, sides or back, you may find it quite hard to apply a bandage. There are a couple of shortcut techniques you can employ until you get your pet to the vet.

By far the simplest is to slip your pet's front legs through the arms, and their head through the neck opening, of a clean cotton T-shirt. Then use adhesive tape on the waist around the middle to keep it in place. Take care there are no toxic inks or ingestible adornments such as beads on the shirt that your pet can swallow.

You can make a multi-tailed body bandage with any rectangular length of clean and inert (no printing or adornments) material. What you do is cut several slits on each opposite side of the rectangle to make tie-offs. Depending upon whether the wound is on the back or below the body, use these tie-offs to secure the temporary body bandage to cover the wounded area. However, this style of temporary body bandage can move around when your pet itself moves around or walks.

An actual body wrap, made from an old towel, sheet or similarly sized piece of material is very useful for preventing your pet from scratching or chewing at a body injury.

The easiest way to make one for your pet is to have them stand on the material and mark out the position of the feet when your pet has a comfortable stance standing on it. Moving your pet aside, cut leg holes at the points you have marked. Then gently feed your pet's legs through the holes and elevate the fabric to cover his body. You can then keep it in place along the back with high-quality safety pins. If you need to add foot protection for your dog, you can then attach cotton socks to the body wrap, pulling them up over the feet and securing them to the body wrap with quality safety pins.

Making a splint

For a suspected leg fracture, the ideal response is to get your pet to a vet as soon as you can. However, First Aid requires that you can immobilise the joints both above and below the leg to stop them from moving and doing further damage to the leg. For this reason, you will find that First Aid for a leg bone breakage only works for the bones in the lower legs.

You need to use a splint to pad out and protect the animal's leg from further damage. Ideally, any splint should cover the whole leg. You can make one from any form of rigid material, such as a rolled newspaper, some cardboard, or even a tightly folded towel that you wrap around. However, there is no doubt that for a temporary bone hold, bubble wrap is possibly the best, being both rigid for protection yet soft to the touch at the same time.

Do remember that for bone breakages, all you need to do is hold the bone in place until you can get your pet to the vet.

You really must not attempt a home-applied splint as a fix for a bone fracture.

In use, what you do is, with your pet's weight kept off their suspected fracture, gently place your pet's leg on the material you have chosen for your splint and wrap it carefully around the leg taping it in place. You always do this from the foot, taping upwards toward the animal's body.

You then must then take your pet to the vet immediately to ensure the corrective treatment is applied as soon as possible.

Safe transport

When you are moving your injured pet, as you will have to do a body wrap to get him to the vet (unless your pet is very poorly and your vet will undertake a house visit), you must do so with absolute care and attention. If you don't, you will not only cause your pet pain, but could very well also end up making any problems far worse than they originally were before your intervention.

If there are only minor problems or injuries evident, you may find that your dog wants to walk out to your car by himself. If that is the case, simply let him. However, if your dog is used to jumping into the car boot or onto the back seat, you most certainly must prevent him from doing so.

Even with an injury or an incapacity, he will want to do what he is used to always doing.

Also, it is accepted that injured pets should not be allowed to rest in your arms. Your own upset can actually cause them further upset and you may find that it can affect their breathing too.

You will also find that even for the smallest of pets, they can get heavy in your arms very quickly, and should you need to make yourself more comfortable by shifting to a different position in your seat, if your pet is in your arms, you can cause you them unnecessary extra pain or even further damage.

If the injury is of a much more serious nature:
Ensure broken legs are carefully supported – you may need to splint before moving

- You will possibly need to support your pet's back
- In chest injury situations, if your pet has a lung problem, try to lay your pet with his problem lung downwards and his less or uninjured lung upwards to help ease breathing
- If you can, let your pet find their own most comfortable position for resting and breathing.

Types of transport

When transporting an unwell pet to the vet, there are a few alternatives you can employ to get them there as comfortably and safely as possible without adding extra damage to an existing problem.

A pet carrier cage, basket or box

Smaller pets are best transported to the vet when they can be comfortably kept in a carrier of some description.

This means you can move them from home to car and from car to vet's practice without causing the potential further discomfort or harm that can occur if you shift your position when they are on your lap.

Firm surface board

A firm surface for laying your pet on is almost a must where there might be a back injury involved. Place a board on the floor or ground beside your injured pet and then carefully and gently slide her back-first onto the surface of the board. Do this with one hand beneath her hips and the other beneath her hips.

For a small pet, they can be moved using a large kitchen tray or kitchen cutting board, an easily removable kitchen cupboard door or even a bookshelf.

The bigger pet may need the likes of a sheet of wood, an ironing board or a sheet of plywood. Just double-check that the laden flat board will fit in the vehicle you plan to take your pet to the vet practice in.

You will need to also use a blanket or towel to cover your pet on the board as well as tape, belts, leg stockings or something similar ensure your pet doesn't slip off in transit.

What you use to keep your pet safe on the journey is placed over the body just behind the front legs and in front of the hind legs. Don't forget that the tie-downs are placed over the blanket or towel.

You will of course appreciate that for the larger dog, you will need two people, one at each end, to carry the board flat and into the car.

Temporary stretcher

If you don't have a board to hand, or you haven't one big enough for a large dog, or for that matter, your car won't accommodate a large board, you can place your pet on a (double-folded) blanket or towel for two people to carry, one at each end, like a stretcher. Just take care not to let the improvised stretcher sag too much in the centre under the weight of your pet as this may end up doing further damage.

Some basic follow-up care

As you will have no doubt learned by now, First Aid is simply what it "says on the tin", namely solely the very first care required to see that an injury is treated. So that your pet will heal correctly and recover back to best health, you will find that, like it is for humans, follow-up care might be necessary for anything from just a couple of days to weeks. It does tend to be just an extension of the care you initially provided with your First Aid. It usually comprises of:

1. Monitoring the progress of the wound healing
2. Cleaning the injury
3. Changing bandages regularly and methodically
4. Giving any vet-prescribed medicines as required, orally, topically or applied or by injection.

Giving liquid medications

Pets do not want to take medicine. Even when it's flavoured. However, there is no doubt that the presentation of liquid medicine to your pet is by far the easiest way.

When prescribed by a vet and from an animal specialist, you will find that many of the oral medicines will come with a syringe with no needle. You 'draw up the correct amount into the syringe and simply place the tip of the syringe into your pet's mouth, slowly squirting the medicine into the cheek. However, you may also need to just dispense a few drops at a time, especially with the cleverer pet! By keeping your pet's head up, gravity will do most of the work for you. You can also gently stroke your pet's throat until the medicine is swallowed. If you don't have a syringe, you can also consider using an eyedropper instead. Make sure any syringe ore eyedropper is 100% clean.

Taking pills

You will find that dogs, especially those in the Labrador, Weimaraner and hunting dog category can be rather greedy at the best of times and will often take any required pills without any bother when cunningly concealed by their owner in their favourite treat. However, some dogs, and certainly most cats will always, no matter how hard you try, swallow the treat and then just spit out the medicinal pill.

You have to ensure your pet does swallow the medicine, otherwise they simply will not benefit end it not only becomes a waste of time but prolongs the length of any sickness.

There is a tried and tested method of dispensing a pill to your dog. Gently, but firmly, grab the top of your dog's snout with your leading hand and press both sides of the jaw in just behind the large, pointed teeth (the canines) along the gum line.

This will make your dog open their mouth wide. You can then sneakily, if you are quick about it, pop any pill over the dog's tongue with your other hand. Slowly let your dog close their mouth and then stroke the throat gently until the dog wallows the pill. Have a treat to had that you can quickly give the dog, so they forget about the pill and therefore doesn't spit it out.

You can try the same with a cat, but they tend to less predisposed to you grabbing them around the nose. If you can't manage, gently grasp the loose fur around the top of the scruff of your cat's neck pulling the head back until the cat's nose points upwards.

You will find at this stage the cat's mouth will simply fall open so you can use a finger to gently pull the jaw downwards and pop the pill – which you should consider coating with some butter or margarine to make it slide down more easily - towards the back of the mouth along the natural channel of the cat's tongue. You can then let the cat close its mouth, keeping an eye out for it to swallow the pill.

You will find that a cat will generally lick its nose after it has swallowed a pill. Alternatively, if you find you are not getting far with having your cat take a pill, you can always crush it into a powder and then mix it into some very strong-smelling cat food at feeding time.

Putting medication on your pet's ears

You will find that your pet has a very long and curved ear canal. As a result, you will have to adopt some special methods to ensure the medicine is applied where it needs to be.

You will find that ear medication is often a topical product in that it will be either an ointment or liquid.

To get the medication to where it has to go, you firstly need to tip your pet's head in the direction that ensures the affected ear is pointing upwards, because that way you can employ the help of gravity.
Drop the required dose of medicine down into the ear canal. Firmly, but gently, take hold of your pet's earflap with one hand to prevent him from shaking his head and the ear drops going all over the place. Use your other hand to gently massage the lower part of the ear. You should hopefully hear the medicine squishing through the inner ear canal.

Putting medication in your pet's eyes

As is the case for your pet's ears, eye medication is more often than not a topical product in that it too will be either an ointment or liquid, and you apply either in the same way as you would for ear medication. Tip your pet's head in the direction that ensures the affected eye is pointing upwards. Pull down the lower eyelid of the appropriate eye very gently, and either squirt or drip the required drops of the medicine into the cupped tissue of the eye. You can then allow your pet to blink several times which will spread the medicine naturally over the surface of their eye.

Bandaging and treating your pet

Injuries to the paw
Place a clean gauze pad over the wound.

Run a strip of gauze from a roll, folded over in half, from the front part of the foot, over the paw and then under the toes.

Starting at the toes, wrap a single strip of gauze all around the paw moving upwards until all the gauze underneath is covered.

The bandage will need to breathe, so preferably using a piece of sticky bandage tape, secure the top part of the bandage only.

Then, put a clean white sock over the entire foot and tape it up at the top.

The wrapping, while ideally it should be firmly applied, shouldn't be too tight. If you can just slip a pencil in between the bandage wrapping and the foot without having to push it in, you know you're OK.

Injuries to the tail

The best method to use to protect a dog's injured tail is a criss-cross mummy wrap.

Firstly, put a cotton tube sock over the tail.

Then, wrap the medical tape around the outside of the sock in the criss-cross mummy-wrap pattern, starting at the tip of the tail and working back towards the body.

Continue with the wrap for at least 5cm past the end of the sock to secure it to the dog's fur at the top of the sock, then wrap back, still in a criss-cross fashion, towards the tip of the tail.

As will be the case for all bandaging, make sure you don't wrap too tightly and make it uncomfortable for your dog.

Injuries to the ear

Firstly, put a piece of gauze pad over the wound.

Gently fold the earflap of the injured head over the top of the dog's head.

Then fold the other earflap over the first one to form a "cap" on the top of the dog's head.
Wrap some gauze or soft fabric cut into a long strip around the dog's head and neck to hold the folded ears in place.

Then tape the bandage in place.

A temporary body bandage

A body bandage can be made from any clean piece of rectangular material such as an old sheet, pillowcase or T-shirt.

Cut parallel slits in each side of the rectangle as straps that you can individually tie over your pet's back.

A temporary body wrap

A body wrap does not only help protect a pet injury but also prevents your pet from either scratching or chewing at the injury.

Stand your pet in as comfortable a stance as possible on whatever material you are using as a wrap and mark the position of the animal's feet. You may have problems in getting a cat to stand, so hover just over the material allowing the cat to dangle its feet as if to stand.

Remove your pet and cut out holes where you have marked the feet positions.

Place your pet back on the cloth, then pull it up over the legs, and contain it at the top with quality safety pins.

If there is an injured leg or paw, put your pet in the body wrap, then cover the limb with a sock. Attach the sock to the body wrap with safety pins so that they can't pull it off.

Administering liquid medicine

To give liquid medicine to your pet, first, tilt the head upright.

Insert either a needleless syringe or an eyedropper into the corner of the mouth and squirt the medicine into the mouth.

Stroke the pet's throat reassuringly until the medicine is swallowed.

Administering a pill

To give a pill to your pet, squeeze their lips gently but firmly against the sides of their teeth.

Once you open their mouth, place the pill on the back of their tongue.

Close the mouth and stroke the pet's throat reassuringly until the medicine is swallowed.

The pill syringe

If you have a pet who you feel may try to take your finger off instead of the pill you are attempting to administer, it could be a worthwhile investment to purchase a pill syringe dispenser, often referred to as a pill gun.

They are available from most pet stores or online.

It is an easy-to-use plastic dispenser you can use to make it simple to dispense a pill into an otherwise unwilling pet's mouth.

Place your pet on a table or countertop at your mid-body height and place your dominant hand on top of their head. You want to ideally encompass their muzzle with your fingers.

Press the lips back against the teeth behind the canine teeth make your pet open their mouth wide.

With your free hand, place the pill syringe on the animal's tongue with the delivery end of the syringe at the back of the throat but not touching it.

Press the mechanism of the syringe to release the pill at the back of the throat and take the syringe out from the mouth immediately.

Then hold your pet's mouth closed and stroke the throat (or gently blow on the nose) reassuringly to make them swallow.

Applying eye medication

For dosing eye medication, gently pull down your pet's lower eyelid and apply a small amount into the cupped tissue.

There is no need to spread it around as the blinking action of your pet will help distribute the medication around the eye.

Try and keep your pet from pawing at the eye for at least ten minutes to allow the medication to work in.

Applying ear medication

For presenting ear medication, firstly, tilt your pet's head with the affected ear uppermost.

Apply the medication into the ear canal, allowing gravity to assist with it penetrating deep into the ear canal.

Then you need to gently massage the base of the ear to ensure the medication does penetrate deep down.

If you hold the earflap with your other hand, this should help keep your pet still.
Try and keep your pet from pawing at the ear.

Having to immobilise your pet

You will find that some injuries will require you to completely immobilise your pet before transportation to the vet. This is not only for your pet's comfort, but importantly, to prevent further damage to an injury.

Carefully, and without jostling your pet in any way, gently slide your dog or cat onto a board or other rigid object.

Cover your pet with a blanket or towel and use strong tape to secure the fabric covering your pet which also, at the same time, immobilises your pet against sudden movement.

Summary list of symptoms and their potential cause/s

It is fair to assume that you may not at first know what's wrong with your pet. There is no shame in this because firstly, there are so many symptoms to recognise, and secondly, you will most probably lack the experience identifying precisely what the problem is.

The following is a basic checklist and instant guide to potential problems linked to visual symptoms you might see, where you'll be able find that which may be causing the problem and be able to best take action to safeguard the health and well-being of your pet. Certain causal problems such as scorpion and snake bites have been left in this list if you take your pet abroad or find your pet gets into an argument with someone else's accidentally liberated pet scorpion or snake.

This is quite a long list, but easy to reference check. Simply pick the main category the observed problem falls into, then the subhead, and then check the potential problem in the alphabetised list under each subhead. Some of the common symptoms have manifestations very similar to one another, so always observe your pet carefully. Diarrhoea, continual scratching or a loss of appetite, as examples, can each be an identical symptom related to totally different causes.

Appetite and eating

- **Appetite loss**

Anal gland impaction, birthing difficulties/problems, foreign object in the mouth, foreign object swallowed, frostbite, incontinence, inhalation of smoke, mastitis, neck pain, puppy strangles, tick infestation, swelling of the jaw, swelling of the tongue, worms

- **No eating**

Bee/wasp stings, falls, foreign object in the mouth, mouth injuries, mouth sores, neck pain, tooth damage

Behaviour

- **Agitated**

Birthing difficulties, foreign object in the mouth

- **Anxious**

Electrical shock, seizures

- **Biting of flanks**

Birthing problems, localised, inflammation, insect bites

- **Chewing their skin, coat, or tail**

Flea allergy, frostbite, hives, hot spots, insect bites, lick sores, skin infections, splinters, tail infections, toe cysts

- **Confused or seemingly drunk**

Carbon monoxide poisoning, low blood sugar, smoke inhalation, snakebites, ticks

- **Crying when using the litter box**

Constipation, urinary blockage

- **Dazed**

Injury to the head

- **Depressed**

Dehydration, hypothermia, mastitis, shock, ticks, urinary blockage

- **Disorientated**

Ear infections, head injuries, low blood sugar, seizures

- **Drools from mouth**

Foreign object in the mouth, head swelling, mouth injuries, mouth sores, poisoning, scorpion stings/snake bites, toad poisoning

- **Frantic**

Choking, foreign object in mouth, jaw entrapment

- **Head bobbing, shaking or tilting**

Earflap injuries, ear infections, foreign object in-ear, foreign object in the mouth, limping, low blood sugar, neck pain

- **Holding head low or stiffly**

Back injuries, foreign object in throat, neck pain

- **Holding mouth open**

Asthma attacks, foreign object in the mouth, mouth injuries, mouth sore

- **Hyperactive**

Foreign object in mouth, jaw entrapment, poisoning

- **Leaving young pups or kittens**

Birthing problems/difficulties

- **Lethargic**

Anal gland impaction, carbon monoxide poisoning, dehydration, heat stroke, hypothermia, poisoning, puppy strangles

- **Licks themselves excessively**

Airborne allergies, anal gland impaction, flea allergy, hot spots, insect bites, lick sores, tick bites, toe cysts

- **Malaise**

Birthing difficulties, foreign object swallowed, poisoning, smoke inhalation

- **Paddles with legs**

Head injuries, seizures, snakebites

- **Reluctance to stand or walk**

Back injuries, collapses, fractures, heatstroke, ticks

- **Restlessness and/or pacing**

Birthing problems, bloated

- **Rubs their face**

Airborne allergies, food allergies, other allergies

- **Sleepy much of the time**

Head injuries, hypothermia

- **Soils inside house**

Diarrhoea, incontinence, seizures, urinary blockage

- **Stares blankly**

Head injuries, seizures

- **Tires easily**

Back injuries, chest injuries, dehydration, fever, strangulation

- **Tooth grinds**

Constipation, foreign object swallowed, seizures, ticks

- **Tucking-in tummy through pain**

Foreign object swallowed

- **Walks in circles**

Ear infections, head injuries

- **Whines or cries for no particular reason**

Abdominal wounds, birthing difficulties, collapse, constipation, dehydration, ear infections, foreign object in the mouth, heat burns, heatstroke, neck pain, urinary blockage

- **Won't lift or tilt their head**

Back injuries, neck pain

- **Won't move around**

Abdominal wound, collapses, falls, unconsciousness

- **Yelps**

Traffic accidents, hedgehog spines, porcupine quills, scorpion stings

Digestion and elimination

- **Abdominal swelling/potbelly**

Bloated, bowel obstruction, constipation, foreign object swallowed

- **Blood in stools**

Ticks, worms

- **Blood in urine**

Poisoning, urinary blockage

- **Dark-coloured urine**

Poisoning, ticks

- **Diarrhoea**

Bee and wasp stings, carbon monoxide poisoning, eating the wrong food, fading puppy, fever, food allergies, foreign object swallowed, heatstroke, poisoning, worms

- **Difficulty urinating**

Anal gland impaction, rectal prolapse, urinary blockage

- **Sloppy stools**

Diarrhoea, worms

- **Smells to the extreme in stools**

Constipation, diarrhoea

- **Specks in stools**

Worms

- **Stomach pain**

Bloated, bowel obstruction, constipation, foreign object swallowed, overeating, worms

- **Urinates involuntarily**

Poisoning, seizures

- **Urinates less often**

Urinary tract blockage

- **Urinates more often**

Poisoning

- **Urine dribbles or leaks**

Incontinence

- **Urine scalding**

Incontinence

- **Vomits**

Bowel obstruction, carbon monoxide poisoning, food allergies, foreign object swallowed, heatstroke, over-eating, poisoning, urinary tract blockage, worms

Ears

- **Abnormal ear odour**

Ear infections, foreign object in the ear

- **Bleeds from inside**

Traffic accidents, clothes-dryer injuries, falls, head injuries

- **Crumbly black or brown material**

Ear infections

- **Crusty margins and ear tips with leaking serum**

Fly bites

- **Discharge from ear**

Ear infections, foreign object in the ear

- **Drooping ear tips**

Frostbite

- **Inflammation**

Ear infections, frostbite

- **Itching**

Ear infections, insect bites, ticks

- **Loss of hearing**

Carbon monoxide poisoning, ear infections, foreign object in the ear

- **Scratches or paws ears, and also,**
- **Soreness**

Ear infections, foreign object in-ear, ticks

- **Swellings**

Earflap injuries, ear infections, foreign object in the ear

Eyes

- **Bloodshot eyes**

Eye infections, foreign object in the eye

- **Discharge**

Eye infections, foreign object in the eye, sties

- **Eyelid irritation**

Bites from animals, insect bites, sties

- **Eyelid swells**

Bee and wasp stings, insect bites, sties

- **Eyes water**

Foreign object in eye, poisoning

- **Glassy or sunk in**

Dehydration, low blood sugar, shock

- **Gray or blue rim**

Drowning, hypothermia, shock

- **Looks in two different directions (divergent eyes)**

Head injuries

- **Out of socket**

Bites from animals, traffic accidents, eye out of the socket, falls, grabbing prominent-eyed dog (e.g. Pug) too firmly

- **Paws eyes**

Foreign object in the eye, insect bites around eyes, sties

- **Rapid blinking**

Eye infections, foreign object in the eye

- **Redness and itching**

Sties

- **Squints**

Eye infections, foreign object in the eye

- **Tear gland swells**

Sties

Head, mouth, nose, and teeth

- **Ammonia-scented breath**

Incontinence

- **Bad breath**

Foreign object in the mouth, mouth injuries, mouth sores

- **Blood in saliva**

Foreign object in the mouth, mouth injuries, mouth sores, tongue tear, tooth damage

- **Blood in vomit**

Heatstroke, poisoning, worms

- **Bloody nose**

Foreign object in nose, head injuries, heatstroke, nosebleeds, snakebites, ticks

- **Burns on lips, corners of mouth, or tongue**

Electrical shock, attempted intake of very hot liquid

- **Difficulty with swallowing**

Foreign object in throat, sore throat, tonsillitis

- **Drools**

Foreign object in the mouth, head swelling, jaw swelling, mouth injuries, mouth sores, poisoning, scorpion stings, toad/frog/amphibian poisoning, tongue swelling, tooth damage

- **Face droops**

Ear infections, head injuries

- **Facial swelling**

Bee and wasp stings, head swelling, hives

- **Gum stickiness**

Abdominal wounds, bites from animals, bloat, burns from heat, collapse, dehydration, foreign object swallowed, heatstroke, shock, smoke inhalation

- **Gum swells**

Mouth sores

- **Gums, blue**

Drowning, hypothermia, mouth injuries, smoke inhalation, suffocation

- **Gum, bright red**

Carbon monoxide poisoning, heatstroke

- **Gum, dark pink or red**

Heatstroke

- **Gum, grey, white, or pale**

Bee, wasp or other insect stings, bites from animals, bloated, drowning, foreign object swallowed, hypothermia, shock, smoke inhalation, toad/frog/amphibian poisoning

- **Gum, purple**

Asthma attacks

- **Head swells**

Bee and wasp stings, head injuries, head swelling, hives

- **Head trapped**

Head entrapment, jaw entrapment

- **Jaw bleeds**

Fractures, jaw entrapment

- **Jaw swells**

Foreign object in mouth, jaw entrapment

- **Lip lesions (in CATS)**

Mouth sores

- **Lip swells**

Mouth sores

- **Lips, blue or grey**

Drowning, hypothermia, shock

- **Mouth pain**

Mouth injuries, mouth sores, tooth damage

- **Mouth sores**

Jaw entrapment, mouth sores, tooth damage

- **Mouth swells**

Jaw entrapment, mouth sores

- **Mouth wounds**

Foreign object in mouth, jaw entrapment, mouth injuries

- **Nasal discharge**

Foreign object in the mouth, foreign object in nose, nosebleeds

- **Nasal dryness**

Foreign object in nose, jaw swelling

- **Object protruded from nose**

Foreign object in the nose

- **Pawing mouth**

Foreign object in the mouth, mouth injuries, mouth sores, toad poisoning

- **Saliva, thick**

Dehydration, toad/frog/amphibian poisoning

- **Salivates excessively**

Mouth sores, poisoning, toad/frog/amphibian poisoning

- **Tongue or gums, blue**

Asthma attacks, carbon monoxide poisoning, cardiac arrest, smoke inhalation, suffocation

- **Tongue swells**

Bee and wasp stings, foreign object in mouth, mouth sores, tongue swelling

- **Tongue, bright red**

Choking, foreign object swallowed, heatstroke

- **Tongue, pale**

Hypothermia, shock

- **Tooth grinding**

Foreign object swallowed, seizures, ticks

Heart and circulation

- **Bleeding**

Abdominal wounds, bites from animals, bleeding, traffic accidents, chest injuries, cuts and wounds, earflap injuries, fractures, pellet/gunshot wounds, head injuries, shock

- **Erratic heartbeat**

Electrical shock, poisoning, shock

- **No heartbeat**

Cardiac arrest

Rear and tail

- **Anal swelling with redness**

Anal gland impaction, rectal prolapse

- **Bites rear end**

Anal gland impaction, constipation, worms

- **Licks rear end**

Anal gland impaction, rectal prolapse, vaginal prolapse, worms

- **Object protrudes from anus**

Bowel obstruction

- **Odour**

Abscesses, constipation, maggots

- **Pus**

Abscesses, tail infections, urinary blockage

- **Rice-like objects near the tail**

Worms

- **Scoots around on the bottom**

Anal gland impaction, constipation, worms

- **Tail sensitivity**

Anal gland impaction, tail infections, tail swelling

- **Tail soreness**

Tail infections, tail swelling

- **Tail swells**

Tail infections, tail swelling

- **Tissue bulging under the tail**

Birthing problems, rectal prolapse, vaginal prolapse

Legs, hips, and paws

- **Bleeding**

Bites from animals, traffic accidents, fractures

- **Bone protrudes**

Fractures

- **Difficulty getting up**

Falls

- **Drags leg**

Back injuries, fractures, tick bites

- **Holds paw up**

Fractures, ingrown nails, leg swelling, limping

- **Hopping walk**

Falls, ingrown nails, kneecap slipping

- **Inability or reluctance to stand**

Back injuries, fractures, pad burns, paw damage, shock

- **Leg dangling**

Traffic accidents, fractures

- **Leg at an odd angle**

Fractures

- **Leg swells**

Abscesses, bites from animals, traffic accidents, frostbite, ingrown nails, kneecap slipping, leg swelling, limping, nail-bed infections, ticks

- **Licks paws or toes**

Airborne allergies, ingrown nails, nail-bed infections, ticks, toe cysts

- **Limps**

Abscesses, arrow wounds, bites from animals, bleeding, traffic accidents, falls, fractures, frostbite, ingrown nails, kneecap slipping, leg swelling, limping, nail-bed infections, pad burns, paw damage, ticks

- **Loss of use of hind legs**

Back injuries, ticks

- **Pad bleeds**

Ingrown nails, paw damage

- **Pad blisters**

Pad Burns

- **Pad cracks or calluses**

Pad burns, paw damage

- **Pad inflammation**

Ingrown nails, pad burns, paw damage, toe cysts

- **Pad swells**

Ingrown nails, nail-bed infections, paw damage

- **Pad wounds**

Pad burns, paw damage

- **Paw abrasions**

Burns from friction, paw damage

- **Paw burns**

Burns from friction, pad burns, paw damage

- **Paw puncture**

Ingrown nails, paw damage

- **Paw swells**

Nail-bed infections

- **Pus drains from paws**

Nail-bed infections, pad burns, paw damage

- **Stretches leg backwards**

Kneecap slipping

- **Toe soreness**

Nail-bed infections, paw damage, toe cysts

- **Unsteady**

Head injuries, seizures

- **Walks with back toes turned under**

Back injuries

- **Walks stiff-legged**

Birthing problems

- **Walks straddle-legged**

Testicular or scrotal swelling, urinary blockage

- **Wobbly hind legs**

Back injuries, ticks

- **Won't let paw be touched**

Cuts and wounds, ingrown nails, nail-bed infections, paw damage, splinters

Reproductive system

- **Breast hardness**

Mastitis

- **Breast inflamed**

Abscesses, mastitis

- **Breast swells**

Bloat, mastitis

- **Failure to nurse**

Fading puppy or kitten, mastitis

- **Labour without delivery**

Birthing problems

- **Nipple discharge**

Mastitis

- **Reduced milk production**

Mastitis

- **Scrotal swelling**

Frostbite, testicular or scrotal swelling

- **Testicular hardness**

Testicular or scrotal swelling

- **Testicular inflammation and swelling**

Testicular or scrotal swelling

- **Tissue protrudes from the vagina**

Vaginal prolapse

- **Vaginal discharge, malodorous**

Birthing problems

Respiratory system

- **Breath, shortness of**

Burns from heat, carbon monoxide poisoning, collapse, strangulation

- **Breathes noisily**

Asthma attacks, bee and wasp stings, foreign object in the nose, foreign object in the throat

- **Breathes rapidly**

Burns from heat, collapse, fractures, heat stroke, shock

- **Breathes shallowly**

Arrow wounds, chest injuries

- **Breathing difficult or laboured**

Asthma attacks, bee and wasp stings, traffic accidents, chest injuries, choking, collapse, distemper, drowning, electrical shock, falls, food allergies, foreign object in the throat, fractures, pellet/gunshot wounds, head entrapment, hives, poisoning, scorpion sting, smoke inhalation, strangulation, suffocation, ticks, tongue swelling

- **Breathing stopped**

Bites from animals, traffic accidents, cardiac arrest, clothes-dryer injuries, foreign object in the nose, foreign object in the throat, fractures, heatstroke, jellyfish stings, low blood sugar, poisoning, shock, smoke inhalation, snakebites, strangulation, suffocation, toad/frog/amphibian poisoning, unconsciousness

- **Coughs**

Asthma attacks, choking, collapse, electrical shock, foreign object in the throat, kennel cough, pneumonia, smoke inhalation

- **Gags**

Choking, collapse, fishhook injuries, foreign object in the mouth, foreign object in the throat, head swelling, jaw swelling, mouth injuries, mouth sores, poisoning, tooth damage

- **Gasps**

Asthma attacks, carbon monoxide poisoning, foreign object in the throat, smoke inhalation, suffocation

- **Pants (in CATS)**

Birthing problems, heatstroke

- **Sneezes**

Foreign object in the nose

- **Snorts**

Foreign object in the nose, foreign object in the throat

- **Throat swollen shut**

Bee and wasp stings, heatstroke

- **Wheezes**

Asthma attacks, bee and wasp stings, foreign object in the throat

Skin and coat

- **Bite Wounds**

Abscesses, bites from animals, snakebites, spider bites, ticks

- **Blisters**

Burns from chemicals, burns from heat, frostbit

- **Discharge**

Abscesses, burns from chemicals, burns from heat, frostbite, skin infections

- **Flakiness**

Skin infections

- **Fur loss, patchy**

Flea allergy, hot spots, lick sores

- **Fur loss, skin red to grey**

Airborne allergies, food allergies, skin infections

- **Fur, wet and smelly**

Abscesses, diarrhoea, incontinence, maggots

- **Greasiness**

Airborne allergies, skin infections

- **Hives**

Bee and wasp stings, heat, jellyfish stings

- **Inflammation**

Cuts and wounds, suture problems

- **Itches**

Airborne allergies, flea allergy, food allergies, hives, hot spots, impetigo, skin infections, suture/stitching problems

- **Loss of elasticity**

Dehydration

- **Maggots**

Cuts and wounds, maggots

- **Oiliness**

Skin infections

- **Pimples (usually in puppies/kittens)**

Impetigo

- **Pus**

Abscesses, skin infections

- **Rancid odour**

Impetigo, maggots

- **Rash**

Airborne allergies, flea allergy, hives, impetigo

- **Scabs**

Flea allergy, impetigo

- **Skin bumps, red**

Lick sores

- **Skin, blue or grey**

Drowning, frostbite, hypothermia

- **Skin, cold**

Frostbite, hypothermia

- **Skin, hard and nonpliable**

Mastitis

- **Skin, pale or white**

Frostbite, hypothermia

- **Sores**

Abscesses, flea allergy, hot spots, lick sores, puppy strangles

- **Sores, Bull's-Eye**

Skin Infections, ticks

- **Sores, red and shiny**

Skin infections

- **Sores, red and wet**

Abscesses, burns from heat, hot spots

- **Sores, wet and weeping**

Burns from chemicals

- **Splotches**

Airborne allergies, hives, hot spots

- **Swelling**

Abscesses, bee and wasp stings, bites from animals, food allergies, air/gunshot wounds, hives, jellyfish stings, puppy strangles, scorpion stings, skin swelling, snakebites, suture problems

- **Welts**

Hives

- **Worms in wound**

Abscesses, maggots

Whole-body symptom

- **Cold to Touch**

Hypothermia

- **Collapse**

Bee and wasp stings, birthing problems, traffic accidents, collapse, food allergies, jellyfish stings, low blood sugar, poisoning, seizures, scorpion stings, toad/frog/amphibian poisoning, unconsciousness

- **Dizziness**

Ear infections, heatstroke, low blood sugar

- **Elevated body temperature**

Clothes-dryer injuries, fever, heat stroke, seizures

- **Faints**

Asthma attacks, burns from heat, collapse, ear infections, low blood sugar, poisoning, seizures, smoke inhalation, unconsciousness

- **Falls over**

Ear infections, seizures, unconsciousness

- **Fever**

Abscesses, anal gland impaction, bee and wasp stings, fever, puppy strangles, spider bites, ticks

- **Hunched back**

Abdominal wounds, back injuries, constipation

- **Lack of movement**

Collapse, fading puppy or kitten

- **Low body temperature**

Drowning, frostbite, hypothermia, shock

- **Lumps, hard or soft**

Abscesses, mastitis, skin swelling

- **Neck swells**

Abscesses, neck pain, puppy strangles

- **Paralysis**

Back injuries, scorpion stings, ticks

- **Retching**

Choking, foreign object swallowed, heatstroke, ticks, vomiting

- **Seizures**

Birthing problems, carbon monoxide poisoning, electrical shock, head injuries, low blood sugar, poisoning, seizures, snakebites, toad/frog/amphibian poisoning

- **Shakes, shivers, or trembles**

Bee and wasp stings, hypothermia, low blood sugar, snakebites, spider bites

- **Stiffness**

Fading puppy or kitten, poisoning, ticks

- **Unconsciousness**

Asthma attacks, bites from animals, traffic accidents, cardiac arrest, clothes-dryer injuries, fading puppy or kitten, falls, fractures, head injuries, heatstroke, hypothermia, low blood sugar, neck pain, poisoning, seizures, spider bites, strangulation, suffocation, unconsciousness

- **Weakness or wooziness/grogginess**

Abdominal wounds, bee and wasp stings, birthing problems, burns from heat, carbon monoxide poisoning, clothes-dryer injuries, collapse, dehydration, drowning, ear infections, falls, heatstroke, low blood sugar, poisoning, seizures, shock, suffocation, unconsciousness

Emergency procedures

It is outside the scope of this training manual to detail every First Aid procedure for the symptoms previously listed. However, the following is an abbreviated list of actions for some of the more regular problems requiring First Aid that you may encounter daily.

Remember your emergency Triage

If you have a situation where multiple pets are critically involved, it is the animal with the best chance of living that should be attended to first.

Also, small bandages like we use on humans, do not work very well on animals.

Triage is checking your CPR "**ABC's**"

> **A - AIRWAY** - is the airway open?
>
> **B - BREATHING** - is your pet breathing on its own?
>
> **C - CIRCULATION** - can you detect a heartbeat and a pulse?

Birthing problems

Normally, dogs and cats will not have birthing problems. But dog breeds that have large heads and narrow hips, such as bulldogs, as well as older, overweight, or very nervous pets can have more trouble.

And add to this that for all cats and dogs, a first-time mother may not understand what is going on and create difficulties for herself.

So, an interrupted birth can not only become dangerous for the babies who can die, but it can become painful or life-threatening for the mother.

You can help by using First Aid to assist a new mother in difficulty.

But if your pet seems weak, depressed, gnaws at her nether regions in pain, is in labour for around an hour with no birth, yet is having consistent and recurrent contractions, or if there's a black, yellow or bloody vaginal discharge that smells rotten, you will need vet intervention immediately.

Take your dog's temperature - use a sterilised rectal thermometer lubricated with Vaseline. The temperature always falls a degree or so below normal (37.2°C to 39.2°C) approximately 24 hours before labour.

Clip the dog's fur - this is very important for a long-haired breed of dog.

Provide privacy.

Keep a careful eye out for any problems.

Get help if there appears to be no progress after the mother has been pushing for 20 minutes.

Break open the birthing membrane of the mother doesn't do so herself within 30 seconds of the birth.

Cut any umbilical cords and clamp ends if the mother doesn't herself within 2-3minutes of birth.

Call your vet if needed.

Bites from other animals
Pets can not only be bitten by your other pets as well as the pets of strangers, but also by wild animals.

Bites pose a particular problem because a bite from a cat is harder to detect, while the bite from a dog can be deceptive if the dog shakes its victim while biting thus creating further problems such as tearing ligaments, blood vessels or muscles that don't manifest themselves as problems immediately.

If your pet gets bitten, take it to the vet immediately.

If you see a biting attack on your pet in progress, throw water over them all or make a lot of noise rather than trying to separate them, as you may get bitten as well.

Keep in mind the risk of rabies, even if your vicinity is known to be rabies-free.

Check your ABC of CPR – airway, breathing, circulation.

Perform CPR if necessary.

Watch out for shock.

Check and control any bleeding.

Restrain your pet as comfortably as possible.

Seek medical attention.

Protect any visible wounds appropriately and try and check for any less obvious wounds to treat.

Clear and clean the bite areas.

Numb any apparent pain with ice.

Bloating

This tends to be an extremely short-term (sometimes only for minutes!), attentive observance-only and very dangerous condition in terms of First Aid and will generally need vet intervention immediately.

If you own a large dog and live over half an hour's travel away from your vet, it is good practice to have the vet show you in advance what to do in such cases.

Very large dogs, and dogs that gulp their food down, are often prone to bloating where gases build-up and their stomach appears to be swollen. This has to be monitored very closely, because the dog may vomit excessively or even pass faeces by mouth.

However, if this develops into a twisted gut, which is very dangerous, it too will need immediate vet intervention.

The signs are shock, pale gums, cold gums and even collapse because the twisted gut has cut off the blood supply to vital organs.

Bleeding

Check your ABC of CPR.

Using gauze or a clean cloth, apply direct pressure.

Add more gauze or cloth if it becomes too soaked.

Never wipe the wound – otherwise it may start to gush blood again.

Secure with medical tape.

For **pressure points** where blood vessels travel and the previous technique doesn't work:

Lower jaw - place your middle three fingers at the base of the lower jaw just below where the bleeding is.

Windpipe groove - place your middle three fingers on the area where the bleeding is.

You need to release the pressure you are exerting for a few seconds every 10 minutes at most to prevent the blood flow from being cut off internally.

If it's a neck or head pressure point, ensure you don't block the animal's breathing.

Bowel obstruction

This is a strange one that may not always demand First Aid. If you think it's from a small swallowed object (such as a chocolate wrapper being swallowed by a greedy dog), it can be often the case to wait 24 hours and observe if there is an obvious decline in the dog's health and wellbeing. Dogs suffer from this condition more than cats because dogs are more prone to chewing and eating things, such as sticks and bones.

Keep observing your pet.

Encourage your pet to lick and eat petroleum jelly.

If you see the object start to emerge from your pet's rear, wearing surgical gloves, try to remove it, if necessary, lubricating around the object with a liberal smearing of petroleum jelly.

If you see string dangling, **do not pull,** as it may have something attached to it that could tear the insides of your pet – take them to the vet immediately for an x-ray.

Watch out for any signs of shock.

Burns

Check carefully for any shock or symptoms.

Wash any chemical burns very copiously with water.

Apply cool water or a cool compress to any burned area.

Apply a sterile **non-stick** dressing – it **must** be non-stick.

- **Do not immerse in water or ice!**
- **Do not apply butter or ointment!**

Choking

Open the animal's mouth and gently probe from side to side to try and identify if there is a foreign object that can be removed from the immediate airway.

Providing the animal is small enough, you may hold it by the hips with the head hanging down to allow gravity to help dislodge any object.

For the larger animal, wrap your arms around the animal's waist, clasp your hands together to make a fist just behind the first rib and compress the abdomen by pushing up five times. You then alternate this with five breaths (getting any air into the subject is better than none at all) into the animal's air tract.

If you find you have not managed to stop the choking, administer a sharp blow to the animal's back in between the two shoulder blades - then repeat the abdominal compressions.

Collapse

This is a state where you will have to call your vet at the same time as try and identify why your pet has collapsed. There can be any number of reasons, and you really will be at pains to identify which one and why an otherwise healthy pet collapses. It could be:

- The ingestion of poison
- Internal bleeding from something like cancer
- Collapsed lung

- Heart/circulatory problems
- Reaction to a bug bite
- Delayed reaction shock (in the case of say chewing electric wires)
- Becoming too cold
- Getting overheated.

Check your ABC of CPR and be prepared to perform.

Help your pet to breathe.

If still breathing and you can detect a heartbeat, administer something sweet.

Keep a check out for shock.

Keep your pet warm if cold.

Cool your pet down if hot (pets can suffer from heatstroke).

Temperatures over 41°C will need immediate vert intervention.

Check for tick bites.

Be on the look-out for any back injury as you will have to move your pet very carefully if so – **see section "Types of Transport" on page 94**

Constipation

Constipation in dogs can be the result of eating grass they cannot digest, bones, or from eating other non-digestible matter that interferes with the normal passing of food through the digestive system. A very furry pet can get mats around their rectum and therefore have mechanical constipation where the opening is physically blocked.

If the rectal area is blocked, restrain your pet, cut the fur away and use a warm water rinse and try to soften the matter around the rectal exit.

Do not assume that a straining pet or one visiting the litter tray often and doing nothing is simply constipated. It could be a urinary problem or urinary blockage and is certainly more prevalent in cats. This is an emergency needing immediate medical attention because if the bladder is full, urine can back up to the kidneys and cause irreversible damage.

Pets who exhibit severe constipation, where the faecal matter has hardened within their bodies, may stop eating, have very painful stomachs and may retch and vomit. They will need immediate vet intervention.

Diarrhoea

There are three very important observances to make:

- Diarrhoea present for any time longer than a week (at most) cannot be helped with First Aid
- What you think is diarrhoea could be **inflammatory bowel disease** which needs veterinary intervention for an internal examination and a potential course of drugs and a change in diet
- It could be the sign of something more serious such as **parvovirus or distemper.**

Otherwise, while completely off-putting by the nature of what it is, diarrhoea is extremely common in both dogs and cats and tends to be caused by the pet eating something it shouldn't, whether old rancid food or food that is unsuited to its digestive system, or such irritable such as a chilli or curry.

Withhold food from a pet adult for up to 24 hours to give the digestive system a rest.

Make sure your pet drinks plenty of water, as it could become dehydrated, as the continual evacuation of watery stools removes dramatic amounts of liquid from the animal's body that need replacing.

Consider using OTC medicines such as Pepto-Bismol to assist until you can get your pet to the vet (but beware of any aspirin-like constituents that are very dangerous to administer to cats).

Embedded foreign items in the body

NEVER REMOVE ANY ITEMS IMPALED IN THE ANIMAL YOURSELF

Roll up some gauze or similar material that you can use to hold the item in place in the precise position where it is impaled in the body.

Use either tape, if the item is small enough, or something that fits over the item that can make a brace to ensure the impaled item remains still.

If the item is anyway long (for example a small branch the animal may have stabbed itself with), try to make it shorter without moving it about, or removing it from, the wound – you may need a second pair of hands to steady it while you do this, but if you do judge that there may be some movement if you try to shorten it, do not do so.

Get veterinary assistance as soon as possible.

Fishhooks - never pull or cut the line!

If you can safely do so without aggravating the wound, push the hook through the exit wound.

Use a wire cutter to cut the barb off.

Carefully pull the hook out from the direction that it entered the skin.

The injury should then be treated like a wound.

If when performing any of the above there is an excess of blood, stop and seek vet advice immediately. You should box off the hook so that the animal can't claw it or you don't lay the animal down on the injury if you have to attend the vet.

Eye injury or foreign object/s in the eye

If you detect swelling, squinting or pawing at the eye, or can detect an obvious foreign object, very gently wash the eye with large amounts of tap water or sterile eyewash.

Examine the eye closely to confirm that all of the object/objects has/have been removed from the eye.

Eye displaced out of eye socket

Flush the entire eye carefully with sterile eyewash.

Cover the eye with a moistened non-stick gauze.

Cover over the opposite good eye.

Do not put a lead or restraint around the animal's neck.

Seek immediate veterinary attention.

Fractures

Wash the immediate area with saline solution or clean water if you can see that a piece of bone might be protruding.

Place a sterile dressing very loosely over the wound.

Wrap the dressed wound with medical tape.

If you can't keep the animal completely still for transport to the vet, you will need to apply a splint. You need to lay something rigid along each side of the fractured limb (you can use a couple of pencils if it's a small break, some tightly rolled paper or a tightly rolled (clean) tea towel for a larger animal).

Fix this in place with tape along with several places along the length of the splint, but ensure it includes the joints (if any) both above and below the observed fracture and that it is not wrapped too tightly, as this can potentially cause more damage to the fracture.

If your pet struggles against your efforts, or you can otherwise take it to the vet in a box or pet carrier, and don't splint.

You may also find that sedation is prescribed to help the initial fracture stabilisation process, the animal may have to endure a set period of totally limited movement.

Heatstroke

Typified by the following symptoms:

Body temperature 40°C or above.

Capillary refill time can be either prolonged or very quick.

Collapse.

Excessive salivation.

Heart rate increased.

Laboured or very fast breathing rate.

Mucous membranes appear red.

Vomiting or blood in diarrhoea.

Relocate the animal to a cool or shaded area.

Soak in, or with, cool (**but not iced**) water.

Place towels around head, neck, abdomen and feet.

Discontinue cooling once the temperature reaches 39.4°C.

Incontinence

There are several attributes connected with incontinence in pets, some of which are not medically related.

Some pets urinate to get attention, others can't help it when they get excited, for example, seeing someone they recognise who normally pays them a lot of attention.

Older dogs, like older humans, sometimes can't help themselves as their relevant bladder muscles become looser with age.

Sometimes incontinence can be a result of urinary tract infections, blockages, metabolic problems and sometimes prostate disease.

However, it has been identified that 10% of dogs and 30% of cats over 15 years of age can have kidney disease and unless treated it could lead to kidney failure.

Keep any incontinent animals clean, especially if older.

Use a protective barrier cream to stop urine burns to the skin.

Use an antibiotic cream if necessary.

Check for parasites (especially during the summer months when they are attracted to urine-caused sores) and take appropriate action to eliminate them.

Use suitable plastics and/or pads to protect your domestic flooring/pet's bed and make it more comfortable for your pet during the night.

Leg swelling

While dogs, like humans, can develop cellulitis that causes their leg to swell, cats tend to get swollen legs from bites by other cats that become infected. Dogs, especially the more active breeds, can also see their legs swell from a bruise or accident causing an internal haematoma. There is also swelling caused by insect bites, overlooked breakages or bone cancers and even overlooked dietary problems such as diabetes.

You need to carefully observe your pet and if they consistently won't put weight on the swollen leg, or if your pet isn't eating or drinking as normal and still imping after 48 hours, you need to take your pet to the vet as it could be a fracture.

Also, be aware that swellings can also be a result of heart failure, liver or metabolic disease that will need immediate vet intervention upon its discovery.

If the swollen leg shows no other symptoms and the pet seems otherwise happy, use a cold compress to help with the swelling for 10 to 20 minutes several times a day.

If the pet has arthritis, dose with a buffered aspirin (**but not to cats**).

If the swelling is abscess-related (the swelling will feel hot to the touch) use a **hot** compress several times a day for about four minutes on, four minutes off until the compress cools (**but not in the groin or armpit area**).

If you know it is something like a splinter or an infection from a cut, use an Epsom Salts soak.

For a swelling related to an allergic reaction, administer an antihistamine, following either the printed pack or vet directions.

Limping

Limping can be symptomatic of a serious injury such as a dislocation or a bone fracture. They can also limp following strain or sprain, a bruise, a thorn in the foot, spilt footpad, an overweight dog hurting itself doing a simple thing such as stair climbing, an abscess or a bite wound. Any limp that lasts longer than 24 hours required veterinary intervention.

Hold your pet still.

Treat with a cold compress.

Check with your vet about offering buffered aspirin (**but not for cats**).

Use a hot compress (**but not in the groin or armpit area**) where there is an abscess.

Diagnosing a limp - some common reasons your pet may limp.

Dislocations and fractures: cause severe pain; flesh may be bruised and discoloured; leg may appear odd and/or deformed.

Spinal cord/nerve injuries: occur gradually with degeneration, but at least there is no pain.

Areas of infection: very tender and red. Feel hot, often with breaks in the skin from teeth or claws. Limping can worsen over time accompanied by a fever from the infection.

Sprains and strains: are sudden but will improve without treatment. Pain is mild, pet may have leg limited leg use.

Ricketts: transmitted by bites from ticks can also cause limping.

Lyme disease: causes joints to gradually swell. Lameness may come and go but will need long-term antibiotic treatment.

Arthritis: and other degenerative joint problems develop very gradually, generally with only mild pain and stiffness. The limp can subside as the joint warms up through use.

Near to drowning

Check the ABC's of CPR.

If the animal is unconscious, hold it upside down and allow water to come out of the airway (nose or mouth).

Use CPR as needed.

Treat for shock (keep the animal warm and quiet).

Puncture wound and lacerations

Remove any foreign object, providing it is only small.

Add one teaspoon of salt to a quart of warm water and wash the area with saline.

Dry the area.

Apply bandage.

or

Check ABC's of CPR if necessary.

Check for shock.

Clip the hair around the wound area.

Apply sterile lubricant to the area to keep hair out of the wound.

Flush with saline solution.

Dry the area.

Apply a bandage.

Sedation may be needed for deep or large wound care.

Seizures

The ingestion of poisons and other causes can result in animals having seizures.

Protect the animal from harm if seizing in cluttered surroundings.

- **Do not put your hand in the mouth of, or try to pull on the tongue of a pet having a seizure.**

If you receive professional advice to induce vomiting, use household (3% strength maximum) hydrogen peroxide orally (animals only!).

One teaspoon per 4½ kilos of body weight.

This can be repeated every 20 minutes for three to four doses.

- **Ipecac should not be used for cats or dogs, despite some saying it is safe for medium/big dogs. It is not and can cause, amongst other problems, heart/circulatory problems.**

Skin infections

In humans, the skin is the body's largest organ, and the same also applies to other animals. It is the one organ that is under constant attack from parasites, bacteria, puncture wounds, fungi, poison substances and more. While both cats and dog can easily get skin infections, dogs tend to be more prone to them.

You will notice a skin infection by the attention your pet gives it, such as constantly scratching, biting and licking. Other visual signs are more obvious such as redness, oiliness, flakiness and potential hair/fur loss. You may also find scabs, oozes or just a bad smell. While medical intervention is the best, First Aid can help greatly to decrease the discomfort for your pet. More seriously (but curable by your vet), skin infections can often manifest as a result of a hormone imbalance, either too much hormone present or too little.

Consider muzzling your pet so as not to get bitten (as a defence mechanism) should you treat a sore spot.

Clip the fur away from around and just beyond the infected area.

Thoroughly wash and clean the infected area (or completely immerse your pet if all over – 2.5% benzoyl peroxide added) using **cool water**, as hot or even warm water makes the irritation worse for your pet.

Administer antihistamine.

Snakebite

Only three types of snake are found in the wild here in the UK, so this is not a major problem.

The adder is the only venomous snake of the three.

You should always get a snake bite checked out as soon as possible, as there could be venomous pet snakes that may have escaped domestically. Telling the vet the colour and pattern of the snake that bit your pet could help them treat it more efficiently.

Use the ABC's of CPR.

Check for any shock.

Keep as still and calm as possible (carry the animal).

- **Do not cut the wound or suck the venom.**
- **Do not apply ice or a tourniquet.**

Seek medical attention as soon as possible.

Toxin ingestion

Check for any signs of possible toxin ingestion.

Observe any vomiting or diarrhoea and check for blood.

Observe any seizures or abnormal mental state (see if the dog is hyperexcitable, depressed).

Note any excessive salivation.

See if there are ulcers in the mouth and check for any bleeding from the mouth or any other body cavity.

Check the ABC's of CPR.

Check the mucous membrane colour, the capillary refill time and the animal's mental state.

Check the surroundings for possible further laying poison or toxin.

Unconsciousness

When the blood flow to the brain is interrupted, or the nervous system is prevented from going about its normal business, your pet can fall unconscious, which is generally a medical emergency for your pet. This can also be the case where the brain is not receiving enough oxygen or blood sugar. First aid can assist with preserving your pet's life until you can obtain emergency help.

There are several occurrences that can render your pet unconscious:

Being hit by traffic

Body temperature extremes

Choking

Diabetes

Drowning

Fall from a height

Kidney failure

Metabolism poisoning

Poisoning.

Remove any collar to avoid potentially interfering with breathing.

Check ABC's of CPR if necessary, to check for breathing and heartbeat.

Lift your pet's heat above its body to help with blood flow and breathing.

Keep a regular check for any vomiting.

Do not move your pet around too much trying to keep it as still as possible during transport to the vet.

Special situations to be aware of

Carbon monoxide poisoning/smoke inhalation

Move pet into fresh air immediately – this may be all that is required to revive.

Drowning

Hold pet upside down and very gently shake for 10 seconds. If you have help to hold the pet, thump sharply on both sides of the body.

Electric shock

Disconnect electrical source.

Extreme cold exposure

Make sure pet is dry, wrap in a blanket, administer CPR if necessary, take to vet.

Extreme heat exposure

Ensure the car is cool, take some wet clothes and place your pet near to air vents to help encourage evaporation. You can use ice but only on top of a cloth and not directly on the body.

Heartbeat but no breathing

Artificial respiration will be needed. Make sure the airway is clear.

No heartbeat and no breathing

Artificial respiration along with CPR.

Seizures

Wrap the pet in damp and cold towels and turn on air conditioning in the car for transportation to the vet.

Shock

Gums will become very pale. Can kill in eight to 20 minutes so wrap the pet in a blanket to keep warm and take it straight to the vet.

Throat obstruction

Look inside the pet's mouth and attempt to remove or use Heimlich manoeuvre.

Vomiting

Vomiting can be a very common occurrence with pets, and if you find it happens just once and your pet seems fine afterwards, it should not be of too much concern, but do keep a close eye on it.

But if more than once, or worse, for a couple of days in a row, and this can be dangerous, as it can leave your pet not only dehydrated, but rather poorly.

If your pet continues to vomit, you must seek veterinary attention immediately, and a check-up even if your pet only vomits a couple of times a month.

Remove feeding dish.

Replenish water but only sparingly – offering an ice cube to lick is a good idea.

Treat hairballs for cats.

Administer a mild peptic preparation for dogs, once or twice a day for a day.

Kaopectate can be given to cats once every six hours **for one day only**.

Death

Death, sadly, must be confronted if First Aid is not possible in time or you cannot get the animal to the vet.

The following checks can be performed for several minutes.

Lack of heartbeat - a pulse will normally not be present under such circumstances.

Lack of respiration - this may be irregular in an unconscious animal.

Cardiac standstill via intracardiac injection.

Lack of the blink reflex referred to medically as the corneal reflex. This is an involuntary blinking of the eyelids prompted by stimulation of the cornea (such as through touch or a foreign item), although this could be the result of a peripheral stimulus.

Lack of movement for hours.

The ill-fated presence of rigour mortis.

Closing thoughts

In an emergency, remember your own safety is of the utmost importance.

Prevention and preparation are vital.

Sometimes treating injured animals may not be an option.

THIS BOOK IS WHAT IS SAYS IN THE TITLE, "FIRST AID". IT IS NOT A REPLACEMENT FOR PROFESSIONAL VET TREATMENT

<u>NEVER HESITATE TO CONTACT YOUR VET</u>

DETAILED REFERENCE INDEX

A & D ointment 18
ABC (for CPR) 78, 82, 130-133, 136, 144-148
Absorbent pad 86, 90
Acupuncture Resuscitation 81
Airway, Breathing, Circulation 132
Anbesol 152
Antacid emulsion 10
Anti-flea spray 10
Antifreeze 56
Antihistamine 10, 18, 143, 146
Antiseptic 11, 12, 18-20, 152
Appetite loss 106
Artificial respiration 40, 73, 74, 78, 149
Arthritis 45, 144, 152
Aveeno 18
Bandaging techniques 85
Behaviour 106
       Agitated 106
       Anxious 106
       Biting flanks 106
       Changes 64
       Chewing self 51, 85, 92, 101, **106, 134,** 136
       Confusion 106
       Crying 106
       Dazed 107
       Depressed 38, 42, **44, 107**, **131,** 147
       Destructive 50, **51**
       Disorientated 107
       Drooling 28, **107, 114**
       Excessive self-licking 108
       Frantic 107

Holding head low 107
Hyperactivity 107
Leaving offspring 107
Lethargic 44, **108**
Malaise 108
Mouth open 39, **107**
Paddles legs 108
Pain indicators 19, **27,** 28, 45, 106-110, 116, 128, 129, 131-137, 143, 144
Reluctant to stand/walk 42, **108, 119**
Responsive 41
Rubs face 108
Sleepy 42, 44, **108**
Soils inside house108
Stares blankly 42, **108**
Tires easily 108
Tooth grinding **109, 117**
Tummy tucking 109
Walks in circles 42, **109**
Whines 109
Won't move head 109
Yelps 27, **109**
Benadryl 18
Benzocaine 28
Betadine 18
Bleeding 28, 82-88, **117, 119,** 132-**135**
Bloating **132,** 133,
Bowel obstruction 109, 110, 118, **134**
Breathing/respiration 136,
Breathing problems 122, 123, **130, 140**, 148, 149
Bubble wrap 10, 92
Bufferin 19
Burns 28, 109, 114, 119-129, **134,** 156

Burow's solution 19
Caladryl 19
Capillary refill 24, **33, 140,** 147
Carbon monoxide 35, **106, 115**
Cardiac pump technique 79
Cardiopulmonary Resuscitation (CPR) 11, 37, 63, **73, 78-82**, 130-133, 136, 144-149
Cars 7-8, 51, 55-56, 60, 75, 93, 95-96, 149
Chains and tethering 50-50
Chest and shoulders 32, 65, 69, 74-81, 108
        Wounds 90, 94, 117, 123
Chocolate 53, **56**, 134
Choking **107, 117,** 123, 128, **135**, 148
Cleaning wounds 83, 96
Cling film 10
Collapse 108-109, 114, 122-123, **127**, 128-129, 133, **135, 140**
Collar **60,** 62, **69-70,** 90, 148
        Elizabethan (lampshade) collar 69
Colour of skin/gums 24, **34**
Constipation 10, 19, 106, 109-110, 117-118, 128, **136-137**
Cords and wires 61
Cortaid 19
CPR **78, 82**, 130-133, 136, 144-148
Death 73, **151**
Dehydration test 24, **35**
Diarrhoea 21, 53, 66, 105, 108, **110**, 125, **137**, 140, 147
Digestion and elimination
        Abdominal swelling 109
        Blood in stools 109
        Sloppy stools 110
        Specks in stools 110

       Stomach pain 110
       Vomits 21, 53, **110,** 128, 133, 137, 140, 147, **150**
Dislocations 143
Domestic machinery 59
Dosages of medicines 17
Drowning 144, 149
Dulcolax 19
Ear drops 10, 99
Ears 111
       Abnormal odour 111
       Bleeds from inside 111
       Crumbly black material 111
       Crusty margins 111
       Discharge 111
       Drooping tips 111
       Hearing loss 112
       Inflammation 111
       Injury 89-90
       Itching 111
       Medicating 98
       Ringworm 63
       Scabies 65
       Scratching at 112
       Seepage 28
       Soreness 112
       Swelling 112
Electric shock 66, 149
Elizabethan (lampshade) collar 69
Embedded objects in body 138
Empty bottle 11
Epsom salts **20,** 143
Extreme cold 149
Extreme heat 149

Eye drops 10
Eyes 112
        Bloodshot 112
        Discharge 112
        Eyelid irritation 112
        Glassy 112
        Gray/blue rimmed 112
        Itching 113
        Looks two directions 113
        Medicating 99
        Out of socket 113
        Pawing at eyes 113
        Prominent 68-69
        Rapid blinking 113
        Redness 113
        Seepage 28
        Squints 113
        Sunken 112
        Swelling 112
        Swelling tear glands 113
        Watering 112
Feeding your pet 53
Fencing 49, 51
Fever 45, 64, 108, 110, 127, **128,** 144
Firm surface board 79, **95**
Flea powder/spray 10
Fractures 28, 108, **115,** 117-**119**, 123, 129, **139**, 143
Gauze 20, 84, **86-90**, 99-101, 133, 138-139
Glucose 10
Heart rate 24, **36-37**, 140
Head, mouth, nose, teeth
      Ammonia breath scent 113
      Bad breath 113

Blood
      In saliva 114
      In stools 109
      In urine 109
      In vomit 114
      Vomiting blood 140
Difficulty swallowing 114
Drooling 28, **107, 114**
Face droops 114
Face swollen 114
Gums
      Blue 115
      Bright red 115
      Dark Pink 115
      Gray, white, pale 115
      Purple 115
      Red 115
      Stickiness 114
      Swollen 114
Head trapped 115
Jaw swollen 115-116, 123
Lips
      Blue or gray 115
      Burns on 114
      Lesions (cats) 115
      Swells 115
Mouth
      Administering medication 102-103
      Burns 114
      Drooling 114
      Holding it open 107
      Pain 18, 28,
      Sores 114-116

        Swells 116

        Wounds 116

    Nose

        Bloody 114

        Discharge 116

        Dryness 116

        Object protrudes 116

        Snorts 124

    Pawing of mouth 116

    Saliva

        Bloody 114

        Excessive 116

        Thick 116

    Tongue

        Blue (or gums) 116

        Bright red 117

        Burns on 114

        Drools and swelling 114, 116, 123

        Grinding

        Pale 117

Heart and circulation

    Bleeding 117

    Heartbeat Erratic 117

    No heartbeat 117

Heatstroke 114, **115**, 117, 123, 124, 127, 128, 129, 136, **140**

Heimlich manoeuvre **75**, 150

Hips and flanks 91

Home-made bandage 86-87, 91, 101

Hot compress 29, 142-143

Household cleaners 56, 145

Human medicines **13-21,** 27-28

Hydrocortisone 19

Ice 19, 132, 135, 147, 149-150
ID your pet 158
Immobilising your pet 92, **104**
Incontinence 106, 108, 110, 113, **141**
Insecticides 125
Iodine 18, **20**
Lanacane **20,** 28
Lawn and garden treatments **57**, 59
Legs, hips, paws and pads **88,**118
        Bleeding 118
        Bone protrudes 119
        Can't stand 119
        Difficulty standing up 119
        Doesn't want to stand 119
        Drags legs 119
        Holds paw up 119
        Hopping walk 119
        Leg
                At odd angle 119
                Dangling 119
                Swelling 119
        Licks paws or legs 119
        Limping 107, 119, **143-144**
        Loss of hind leg use 120
        Wobbly legs 121
Lyme disease 144
        Pads (the paw)
                Bleeds 120
                Blisters 120
                Burns 119
                Cracks/calluses 120
                Inflammation 120
                Swellings 120

Wounds 120
Paws **88**
Abrasions 120
Burns 120
Punctures 120
Swellings 120
Pus from paw 120
Stretches leg back 120
Toe soreness 121
Unsteadiness 120
Walking
With back toes inwards 120
Stiff-legged 120
Straddle-legged 120
Won't allow paw be touched 120
Liquid medicines 11, **102**
Liquid paraffin 10
Maalox 20
Meat tenderizer 10
Medications 14, 57, **96**
Mucous membrane colour test 35
Muzzles 71
Temporary 71
Nail clippers 11, 17
Neck 38, 68-70, **90**-91, 109, 128-129, 141
Neosporin 20
Neurological 44-46
Neutering your pet 58
No heartbeat/not breathing 117, 149
Not eating 106
OTC 13, 17, 21, 28, 138
Pain 19, **27**, 28, 45, 106, 107, 109, 110, 116, 128, 129,
131, 135, 137, 143, 144

Pad burns 120
Pepto-Bismol liquid 21
Pet carrier **94**, 140
Pet-proof toys 59-60
Pill syringe 102-103
Plants 160
Pliers 11, 74
Poison 19, 31-32, 35, 42, 46, 49, 55-58, 106-117 (multiple entries), 122-124 (multiple entries), 127-129 (multiple entries), 135, 145-149 (multiple entries)
Preparation H 21
Preventing problems 47
Puncture wounds 146
Respiration 24, **39-40**, 73-77, 78, 149, 151
Responsiveness **22**, 24, **41-42**
Safe transport 93-26
    Cage, basket, box 94
    Firm surface board 95
    Temporary stretcher 96
Saline solution 10, 12, 84, 139, 145
Scabies 161
Scissors 11, 59, 83
Seizures **128-129**, **145**, 147, 149
Shampoo 11
Shock 31-33, 35, 37, 66, 106-107, 112, 114-115, 117, 119, 123, 128-129, 132-134, 136, 144-145, 147, **150**
Skin and coat
    Bite wounds 124
    Blisters 124
    Flakiness 146
    Fur loss
        Patchy 124
        Skin red/grey 125

Wet and smells 125
Greasiness 125
Hives 106, 114-115, 123, **125**, 126-127
Infections 106
    Ears 107, 109, 111-112, 114, 127-129
    Eyes 112-113
    Tail 118
    Leg 119
    Nail bed 120-121
    Pads and paws 120
    Skin 124-126
    Urinary141
    Skin 146
Inflammation 29
    Ears 111
    Pad 120
    Rabies 64
    Skin 125
    Testicular 122
Itching 19-20
    Ears 111
    Head 113
Loss of elasticity 125
Oiliness 125, 146
Pimples 125
Pus
    From paw 120
    Rear and tail 118
    Skin, Impetigo 125
Rancid smell 126
Rash 126
Scabs 65, 126, 146
Skin

Bumps, red 126
Blue or grey 126
Chewing 106
Cold 32, 126
Colour 34
Dehydration 36-37
Flakiness 124
Greasiness/oiliness 125
Hard/non-pliable 126
Infections 146
Injury 29
Itchy 18-20, 125
Lumps 128
Pale or white 126
Pus 125
Red to grey 125
Sores 126
Wounds 83
Splotches 127
Swelling 127
Welts 127
Worms in wound 127
Snake bite 105, **146**
Drools 107
Spinal cord 143
Splint 92-94, 140
Sprains/strains 144
Sterile container 11
Stimulants 58
Styptic powder 11
Rabies **64,** 132
Rear
Anal swelling 117

        Anal redness 117
        Bites rear end 117
        Object protrudes 118
        Odour 118
        Pus 118
        Drags along on bottom 118
        Tissues bulging 118
Reproduction System
        Breasts
                Cancers 59
                Hardness 121
                Inflammation 121
                Nipple discharge 122
                Reduced milk 122
                Swellings 121
        Failure to nurse 121
        Labour no delivery 122, 131
        Testicular/Scrotum
                Hardness 122
                Inflammation and swelling 122
                Swelling 121
        Vagina
                Bad odour 131
                Discharge 122
                Tissue protrudes 122
Respiration 39
        Breathing 24, 31-32, 39-40
                Difficult/laboured 71, 123
                Fast 140
                Gasping 40
                Shallow 40, 123
                Shortness of breath 122
                Stopped 73-77, 123

Wheezes 124
Coughing 123
Gagging 123
Panting (cats) 39, (dogs) 40
Snorts 124
Throat swollen or shut 124
Restraining
Hugging 69
Kneeling 69
Reclining 68
Stretch 68
Ringworm 63-64
Whole body as system
Cold to touch 127
Dizziness 127
Elevated temperature 127
Faints 128
Falls over 128
Fever 128
Hunched back 128
Lack of movement 128
Low body temperature 128
Lumps (hard or soft) 128
Neck swellings 128
Paralysis 64, 128
Retching 128
Seizures 128
Shakes/shivers/trembles 129
Stiffness 129
Unconsciousness 129, **148**
Weakness/woozy/groggy 129
Tail
Pus 118

      Rice-like objects 118
      Sensitivity 118
      Soreness 118
      Swelling 118
      Tissue under bulging 118
Tape 87, 89-91, 100-101, 133, 138, 140
Temperature **43, 45,** 127, 128, 131, 136, 141
      Heatstroke 140
Temporary
      Body bandages 101
      Body wrap 101
      Stretcher 96
Throat obstruction 150
Tobacco 58
Torch 11, 74
Toxic ingestion 56-57, 91
Toys 54, 60
Triage **30-31,** 130
Tweezers 11
Types of transport 94-96
Unconsciousness 31, 40, 109, 123, 127-129, **148**
Urine
      Blood in urine 109
      Dark coloured 110
      Difficulty in urinating 110
      Urinates involuntarily 110
      Urine leaks 110
      Urine scalding 110
      Urinates too often 110
Vicks VapoRub 21
Vomiting 21, 53, 128, 140, 145, 147-148, **150**
Washing soda 11
Weight of your pet 16, 96

Witch hazel 21
Zoonoses 63